Computed Tomography: Physics and Technology

A Self Assessment Guide

Computed Tomography: Physics and Technology

A Self Assessment Guide

Second Edition

Euclid Seeram, PhD, FCAMRT
Active Member, Canadian Radiation
Protection Association

HONORARY ACADEMIC APPOINTMENTS
Adjunct Associate Professor; Medical Imaging and
Radiation Sciences; Monash University, Australia |
Adjunct Professor; Faculty of Science;
Charles Sturt University, Australia |
Adjunct Professor; Medical Radiation Sciences,
Faculty of Health; University of Canberra; Australia

REGULAR GUEST LECTURER
Vision, Compassion, Awareness (VCA) Education Solutions for Health
Professionals Inc., Toronto, Ontario, Canada

WILEY Blackwell

Library of Congress Cataloging-in-Publication Data

Names: Seeram, Euclid, author.
Title: Computed tomography : physics and technology : a
  self assessment guide / Euclid Seeram.
Description: Second edition. I Hoboken, NJ : Wiley-Blackwell, 2022. I
  Includes bibliographical references and index.
Identifiers: LCCN 2022015047 (print) I LCCN 2022015048 (ebook) I ISBN
  9781119819325 (paperback) I ISBN 9781119819349 (adobe pdf) I ISBN
  9781119819356 (epub)
Subjects: MESH: Tomography, X-Ray Computed I Examination Questions
Classification: LCC RC78.7.T6 (print) I LCC RC78.7.T6 (ebook) I NLM WN
  18.2 I DDC 616.07/5722–dc23/eng/20220603
LC record available at https://lccn.loc.gov/2022015047
LC ebook record available at https://lccn.loc.gov/2022015048

Cover Design: Wiley
Cover Images: © Canon Medical Systems Canada Limited

Set in 10/12pt Trade Gothic by Straive, Chennai, India

SKY10035061_070522

Dedication

This book is dedicated with love and affection to Claire and Charlotte, my special, smart, cute, and very witty granddaughters. You bring tremendous joy and happiness to our lives.

Contents

Preface

Computed tomography (CT) has experienced several technical innovations in recent years. For example, iterative reconstruction (IR) algorithms are now commonplace, and all CT scanners offer this technology. Additionally, artificial intelligence–based image reconstruction is now offered by several CT vendors. These algorithms address the problems of the filtered back projection (FBP) image reconstruction algorithm and IR algorithms, especially in low-dose CT examinations. Another important new technical innovation is the photon-counting detector, which offers advantages over current energy-integrating CT detectors. These innovations have all resulted in dose optimization efforts in the care and management of the patient undergoing CT examinations. Dose optimization has become an integral part of CT practice.

This book, *Computed Tomography: Physics and Technology A Self Assessment Guide,* features a wide range of questions focused on topics that address the content requirements of CT physics tnd Technology set by various professional radiologic technology associations, including the American Society of Radiologic Technologists (ASRT), the American Registry of Radiologic Technologists (ARRT), the Canadian Association of Medical Radiation Technologists (CAMRT), the College of Radiographers in the United Kingdom, and professional medical imaging organizations in Africa, Asia, Australia, and continental Europe. Additionally, this book may serve as a resource for biomedical engineering technology programs that include CT systems in their curricula, residents in radiology, and medical physics students studying the use of CT in medical imaging.

Self-assessment questions use the true/false, multiple choice, and short answer formats, as listed for each chapters in the table of contents. These formats are typical of the radiologic technology/radiography organizations listed previously and are characteristic of CT certification examinations.

Enjoy the questions that follow, and best wishes for any examination you take. And remember – your patients will benefit from your wisdom.

Euclid Seeram, PhD, MSc, BSc, FCAMRT
British Columbia
Canada

Acknowledgments

The single most important and satisfying task in writing a book of this nature is to acknowledge the help and encouragement of those individuals who perceive the value of its contribution to the medical imaging science literature. It is a pleasure to express sincere thanks to several individuals whose time and effort have contributed tremendously to this second edition.

The content on which the questions in this book are based is centered around the published works and expertise of several noted medical physicists, radiologists, computer scientists, and biomedical engineers (too numerous to mention here) who did the original research. They are the tacit authors of this text, and I am truly grateful to all of them, in particular Dr. Rob Davidson, PhD, MAppSc (MI), BBus, FASMIRT, professor of medical imaging, University of Canberra, Australia. Dr. Davidson has taught CT physics and instrumentation for decades and provided me with the opportunity to develop a course of studies on CT physics and instrumentation for the Medical Imaging Program at the University of Canberra, Australia. Thanks, mate.

Yet another notable individual to whom I am grateful is Valentina Al Hamouche, MRT, MSc, and CEO of Vision, Compassion, Awareness (VCA) Education Solutions for Health Professionals, Inc. (Toronto, Ontario, Canada). Valentina has given me the opportunity to present face-to-face lectures and live webinars on CT physics and instrumentation and other topics in the radiographic sciences, and I have earned the title Regular Guest Lecturer with her organization (www.VCAeducation.ca). Thank you, Valentina, for bringing continuing education opportunities to students and technologists worldwide.

The people at John Wiley and Sons deserve special thanks for their hard work, encouragement, and support of this project. They include James Watson, senior commissioning editor in health sciences, who accepted the proposal for this work and also provided support to bring it to fruition. Additionally, Anne Hunt and Mandy Collison maintained continuous communications about my writing progress and always offered their assistance on matters relating to this project, and they are to be credited as well. Thank you both. I must also thank the individuals in the production department at Wiley for doing a wonderful job bringing the manuscript to its final form. In particular, I am grateful to members of the production team, who have worked exceptionally hard during the production of this book, especially in the page-proof stage.

I must acknowledge the support and praise I receive from my beautiful family. First, my lovely wife, Trish, is a warm, smart, caring, and very special person in my life. Thanks, babe. Second, my caring and brilliant son, David, and his family deserve special mention for their love, support, and encouragement.

Last but not least, I must thank my students in Canada and all over the world who have diligently completed my CT physics and instrumentation courses at both the diploma and degree levels. Thanks for all the challenging questions, which have always kept me on my toes.

1

Computed Tomography: Pioneering Work and Technical Overview

PRIOR READING ASSIGNMENT

Before attempting to answer these review questions, read the following brief summary notes on this topic.

In radiography, images are usually referred to as *planar images*. These images have the following limitations: superimposition of all structures on the image receptor (film-screen detector) and the qualitative nature of radiographic imaging. The latter simply means that it is difficult to distinguish between a homogeneous object (one tissue type) of non-uniform thickness and a heterogeneous object (bone, soft tissue, and air) of uniform thickness. Furthermore, the beam used in radiography is an open beam (wide beam), and this creates more scattered rays that reach the image and essentially destroy the image contrast.

Computed Tomography: Physics and Technology A Self Assessment Guide, Second Edition. Euclid Seeram.
© 2022 John Wiley & Sons Ltd. Published 2022 by John Wiley & Sons Ltd.

2

Computed tomography (CT) overcomes these limitations by removing the superimposition of structures, improving image contrast, and imaging very small differences in tissue contrast, using a more sensitive detector. In particular, CT produces cross-sectional images of patient anatomy, referred to as *transverse axial images*. These sections are perpendicular to the long axis of the patient. The invention of the CT scanner is credited to two individuals: Godfrey Hounsfield (who worked at EMI [Electric and Musical Industries] in England) and Allan Cormack, who shared the Nobel Prize in Medicine in 1979 for their contributions to the development of the scanner. Both of these pioneers worked out the mathematical solutions to the problem in CT, but Hounsfield is credited with the development of the first useful clinical CT scanner.

The technical evolution of the CT scanner is marked by the development of more efficient data collection methods leading to multislice CT imaging (as opposed to single-slice CT imaging), faster image reconstruction algorithms resulting in low-dose CT scanning, and improved image postprocessing methods such as three-dimensional images.

The major components of a CT scanner include the data acquisition system, the computer system, and the image display, storage, and communications system. The data acquisition system contains imaging system components designed to collect radiation attenuation values from the patient using an x-ray tube and special detectors coupled to detector electronics. These components are housed in what is referred to as the CT *gantry*. The computer is a central and integral component in CT. The primary role of the computer is image reconstruction and image postprocessing. A graphics processing unit (GPU) is now used to reduce the processing requirements of the computer's central processing unit (CPU). Image reconstruction uses special algorithms to create the image using the attenuation values collected from the patient. Today these algorithms are iterative reconstruction algorithms and are much faster than the previous algorithm (the filtered back-projection algorithm).

CT examinations generate large amounts of data; hence large storage space on the order of gigabytes (GB) is required. Storage devices for CT include magnetic tape and disks, digital videotape, optical disks, and optical tape. Communications refer to electronic networking or connectivity by using a local area network or wide area network (LAN or WAN). *Connectivity* ensures the transfer of data and images from multivendor and multimodality equipment according to a defined standard.

A popular standard for medical images is the Digital Imaging and Communications in Medicine (DICOM) standard. CT scanners are now connected to Picture Archiving and Communications Systems (PACS).

In general, the software used in CT includes image reconstruction software, preprocessing software, and image postprocessing software. Image reconstruction software uses algorithms to build up the image from the raw data collected from the detectors. Preprocessing software performs corrections (such as correcting a bad detector reading, for example) on the data collected from the detectors before the data is sent to the computer. Image postprocessing software operates on reconstructed images displayed for viewing and interpretation and typically includes visualization and analysis software.

Self-Assessment Questions will be based on the following Keywords and Concepts

- Major differences between CT and radiography
- Godfrey Hounsfield
- Allan Cormack
- Major components of a CT scanner
- Technical evolution overview
- The imaging system
- The computer system
- Storage capacity
- Connectivity
- CT software

Challenge Questions

Answer the following questions to check your understanding of the materials studied.

True (T)/False (F)

1. CT is a planar radiographic imaging modality.
2. CT was developed by EMI.
3. Godfrey Hounsfield was awarded the Nobel Prize in Medicine for his contributions to the development of the first useful CT scanner.
4. Allan Cormack did not share the Nobel Prize in Medicine with Hounsfield.

4

5. Radiographic imaging produces planar images of the patient's body.
6. CT can show very small differences in tissue attenuation compared to radiography.
7. CT shows soft tissue contrast much better than radiography.
8. CT uses rendering algorithms to create three-dimensional images to enhance diagnostic interpretation.
9. Images produced by the CT scanner are generally referred to as planar images.
10. Two notable technical innovations for CT scanners are the development of multislice detectors and iterative reconstruction algorithms.
11. Data acquisition in CT refers to the process of converting attenuation data to electrical signals that are subsequently converted into digital data.
12. GPUs are now used in CT to reduce the processing requirements of the CPU.

Multiple Choice

1. Which company pioneered the development of the CT scanner?
   A. General Electric Healthcare
   B. Siemens Healthineers
   C. Philips Healthcare
   D. EMI (now called Thorn EMI)
2. Which type of image does radiography produce?
   A. Planar static image
   B. Cross-sectional image
   C. Three-dimensional image
   D. Both A and C are correct.
3. A significant difference between CT and radiography is that:
   A. CT shows very small differences in soft tissue contrast compared to radiography.
   B. CT shows better image sharpness compared to radiography.
   C. CT images show better image contrast than radiographic images.
   D. A and C are correct.
4. Which of the following problems of radiography are overcome by CT?
   1. Superimposition of all structures on the image receptor
   2. The open-beam geometry of radiography, which causes more scattered radiation to reach the image receptor

3. The qualitative nature of radiography
4. The radiographic image receptor sensitivity to radiation
   A. 1 only
   B. 1 and 2
   C. 1, 2, and 3
   D. 1, 2, 3, and 4
5. The major system component of the CT scanner responsible for image reconstruction is the:
   A. Data acquisition components
   B. CT detector
   C. Computer system
   D. Picture archiving and communication system (PACS)
6. Which of the following data sets is used by the CT image reconstruction algorithm to create CT images?
   A. Attenuation data from the patient
   B. Demographic data sets about the patient
   C. Exposure factors (kV and mAs)
   D. The computer storage capacity
7. The anatomical section that is perpendicular to the longitudinal axis of the patient is called the:
   A. Planar section
   B. Transverse axial section
   C. Cross section
   D. B and C are correct.
8. Who developed the first clinically useful CT scanner?
   A. Dr. Euclid Seeram
   B. Dr. Godfrey Hounsfield
   C. Dr. Allan Cormack
   D. B and C are correct.
9. The first CT scanner was limited to scanning only the:
   A. Brain
   B. Chest
   C. Abdomen
   D. Whole body
10. Which of the following recent technical innovations in CT are intended to improve image quality and reduce radiation dose?
    1. Multislice detectors
    2. Iterative algorithms
    3. Dose optimization tools
    4. Quality control tests

A. 1 only
B. 2 and 3
C. 3 and 4
D. 1, 2, 3, and 4

11. The purpose of the data acquisition system components in CT is to:
   1. Produce x-rays
   2. Shape and filter the x-ray beam falling upon the patient
   3. Detect the radiation passing through the patient
   4. Convert the transmitted x-ray photons into digital information
      A. 1 only
      B. 2 and 3
      C. 3 and 4
      D. 1, 2, 3, and 4

12. A term used to describe the transfer of data and images from multivendor and multimodality equipment according to a defined standard is:
    A. Digital Imaging and Communications Standard in Medicine (DICOM)
    B. Connectivity
    C. PACS
    D. Preprocessing of raw CT data

Short Answers

1. What are the basic limitations of radiography that have been overcome by CT scanning?
2. How does CT overcome the limitations of radiography?
3. What major contributions did Hounsfield and Cormack make to the development of the CT scanner?
4. What are the major advantages of CT compared to radiography?
5. What is meant by the term *transverse axial section*?
6. List the major system components of the CT scanner and briefly explain the purpose of each component.
7. Identify notable technical innovations that are intended to improve the imaging performance of the CT scanner
8. Summarize the basic elements of how a CT scanner works
9. Briefly describe what is meant by the term *data acquisition*.
10. Briefly summarize the major purpose of image preprocessing and postprocessing in CT.
11. Briefly explain the meaning of the term *communication* as used in the acronym PACS.
12. Why is a GPU now used in CT scanner technology?

Answers to Challenge Questions

True/False

1. F	5. T	9. F
2. T	6. T	10. T
3. T	7. T	11. T
4. F	8. T	12. T

Multiple Choice

1. D	5. C	9. A
2. A	6. A	10. D
3. D	7. D	11. D
4. D	8. B	12. B

Short Answer

1. The fundamental limitations of radiographic images are the superimposition of all structures on the detector (which makes it difficult and sometimes impossible to distinguish a particular detail) and the qualitative nature of radiographic imaging. The latter simply means that it is difficult to distinguish between a homogeneous object (one tissue type) of non-uniform thickness and a heterogeneous object (bone, soft tissue, and air) of uniform thickness. Finally, the beam used in radiography is an open beam (wide beam), and this creates more scattered rays that reach the image and essentially destroy the image contrast. CT overcomes these shortcomings.

2. CT removes the superimposition of structures by using very highly collimated x-ray beams, hence decreasing the amount of scattered radiation produced in the patient. Removal of scatter improves image contrast. CT also uses more sensitive electronic detectors that can discriminate very small differences in tissue contrast compared with film screen image receptors. While radiographic film can only show x-ray intensity differences between 5% and 10%, CT can detect density differences from 0.25% to 0.5%, depending on the scanner.

3. Both Hounsfield and Cormack shared the Nobel Prize in Medicine in 1979 for their contributions to the development of the scanner. Both individuals worked out the mathematics of CT. While Hounsfield's Nobel lecture was entitled "Computed Medical

Imaging," Cormack's Nobel lecture was entitled "Early Two-Dimensional Reconstruction and Recent Topics Stemming from it." Specifically, Hounsfield developed the first clinically useful CT scanner; that is, images were diagnostic and could be interpreted by a radiologist.

4. The major advantage of CT compared to radiography is that CT shows much better image contrast. While the contrast resolution (mm at 0.5%) of radiography is 10, it is 4 for CT and 1 for magnetic resonance imaging (MRI). Additionally, CT is now a three-dimensional (3D) imaging modality. Using 3D rendering algorithms, CT can transform two-dimensional transverse axial images into several types of 3D images, as illustrated in Figure 2–3 in the textbook *CT at a Glance* (Seeram 2018). These image types are intended to enhance diagnostic interpretation.

5. A transverse axial section is illustrated in Figure 1–4 in *CT at a Glance* (Seeram 2018), and it is defined as an anatomical section that is perpendicular to the long axis of the patient. Such a section removes the superimposition of structures above and below the focal plane of the volume of the patient being imaged.

6. A CT scanner has three major system components: the data acquisition system, the computer system, and the image display, storage, and communication systems. The data acquisition consists of the x-ray tube, detectors, and detector electronics, which collect transmission or attenuation data from the patient. The computer uses the attenuation data collected from points around the patient for at least 360° and special image reconstruction algorithms to create CT images. The latter system components of the CT scanner are intended to display images for viewing and interpretation on a monitor, after which they are stored for retrospective analysis using storage hardware such as optical storage disks. These images are then handled by another system component and can be sent to a different location using computer network communications technology. One popular such technology is a PACS.

7. In brief, CT has evolved from a scanner dedicated to imaging the brain only to a single-slice whole-body scanner and, today, to a multislice scanner (MSCT). Other notable technical innovations includes the development of multislice detectors, iterative reconstruction algorithms, virtual reality imaging methods, dose optimization methods, and important quality control test tools

and procedures. Currently, artificial intelligence (AI) is being applied to CT image reconstruction and other areas. These innovations are intended to improve image quality and reduce radiation dose, and they also play a role in the care and management of the patient during CT imaging.

8. The following summarizes the essential technologies (highlighted in italics) that play important roles in describing how a CT scanner works:

   - The *x-ray tube* and *sensitive electronic detectors* are coupled and rotate around the patient to collect *attenuation data* from the patient, who is positioned on the *CT table* (or *couch*, as it is sometimes called), which moves through the *gantry opening* on the CT scanner during *scanning*. This process is referred to as *data acquisition*.

   - The attenuation data is used by *special computer algorithms* to reconstruct CT images. These algorithms are called *image reconstruction algorithms*. *Image reconstruction* is the heart of the CT scanner. Without this, there will be no transverse axial CT images. The basis for image reconstruction is *mathematics*.

   - Images are *displayed* on a *monitor* for viewing and interpretation by an observer who can apply *image postprocessing* to further enhance image sharpness, brightness, and contrast. Images can be *stored* using *optical or magnetic storage devices*, and they can be sent to remote locations using *computer network technologies*, such as a *PACS*.

9. Data acquisition is the first step in the CT process. It refers to the collection of attenuation data (or x-ray transmission data) as the x-ray tube and detectors rotate around the patient, and the subsequent conversion of this data to electrical signals by the detectors. These signals are then converted to digital data by the detector electronics.

10. *Image preprocessing* and *image postprocessing* ate two categories of software used in CT. The third category *is image reconstruction* software. While the purpose of preprocessing is to perform corrections (such as correcting a bad detector reading, for example) on the data collected from the detectors before the data is sent to the computer, image postprocessing software operates on reconstructed images displayed for viewing and interpretation. Examples include visualization and analysis soft-

ware. Visualization software can provide several image types such as multiplanar reformation (MPR), maximum or minimum intensity projection (MIP), and 3D surface-shaded display.

11. *Communications,* as used in the acronym PACS, refers to electronic networking or connectivity using a local area network or wide area network (LAN or WAN). Connectivity ensures the transfer of data and images from multivendor and multimodality equipment according to a defined standard. A popular standard for medical images is the DICOM standard.

12. Presently, CT scanners use iterative reconstruction algorithms to reconstruct images. These algorithms are complex and require increased computational power. Since current CPUs cannot handle these computations, a GPU is used to reduce the processing requirements of the CPU.

IDENTIFYING AREAS TO STUDY

A. Make a list of topics and/or questions that are still not clear to you after studying this chapter.
B. See the instructor for clarification and/or consolidation of the material.

2

Data Acquisition Principles

PRIOR READING ASSIGNMENT

Before attempting to answer these review questions, read the following brief summary notes on this topic.

The questions in this chapter are based on the basic data acquisition principles of the CT scanner. Essentially, there are two data acquisition methods in CT. The first is *conventional slice-by-slice* or *stop-and-go* technology. The limitations of this approach led to the development of *volume data acquisition*, which has now become commonplace. This method is based on the continuous rotation of the x-ray tube and detectors (made possible by slip rings) and simultaneous translation of the patient through the scanner gantry in order to scan a volume of tissue (rather than one slice) in a single breath hold, resulting in a special beam geometry referred to as *spiral* or *helical geometry*. Additionally, the evolution of these scanners is based on

Computed Tomography: Physics and Technology A Self Assessment Guide,
Second Edition. Euclid Seeram.
© 2022 John Wiley & Sons Ltd. Published 2022 by John Wiley & Sons Ltd.

the beam geometry, the scan motion, and the number of detectors (scan time is inversely proportional to the number of detectors) used on the scanner, as illustrated in Figure 2.1.

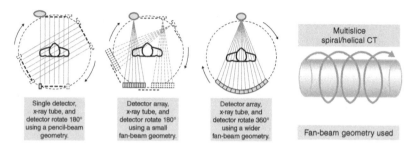

Single detector, x-ray tube, and detector rotate 180° using a pencil-beam geometry.	Detector array, x-ray tube, and detector rotate 180° using a small fan-beam geometry.	Detector array, x-ray tube, and detector rotate 360° using a wider fan-beam geometry.	Multislice spiral/helical CT Fan-beam geometry used

Figure 2.1   **Essential characteristics of four generations of CT scanners.**

The term *geometry* refers to the size, shape, and motion of the x-ray beam and the path it traces as the patient moves through the CT scanner gantry opening during scanning. Furthermore, this geometry is referred to as a *fan-beam geometry* and is characteristic of multi-slice CT (MSCT) scanners. These scanners have developed from 4, 8, 16, 32, 40, and 64 to 320 and now 640 slices per revolution of the x-ray tube and detectors. Two MSCT scanners have been developed specifically for imaging the beating heart: the Toshiba Medical Systems Aquilion CT scanner family (320 slices per revolution of the x-ray tube and detectors) and the Dual Source CT (DSCT) scanner (Siemens Healthcare), designed for cardiac CT imaging because it provides the temporal resolution needed to image moving structures such as the heart.

The major technical data acquisition components of the CT scanner are highlighted in Figure 2.2.

These include the following components: the x-ray tube, x-ray beam filter, prepatient collimators, detectors, and detector electronics (analog-to-digital converters). Each of these plays an important role in accurate imaging of the patient during CT scanning. First, the x-ray tube produces the x-ray beam for the examination, which is in perfect alignment with the detector array. The tube and detector scan the patient to collect a large number of transmission measurements. Second, the x-ray beam is shaped by a special filter as it leaves the

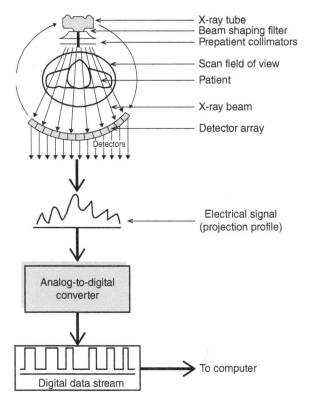

X-ray tube
Beam shaping filter
Prepatient collimators
Scan field of view
Patient
X-ray beam
Detector array
Detectors
Electrical signal
(projection profile)
Analog-to-digital
converter
To computer
Digital data stream

Figure 2.2 The major technical data acquisition components of a CT scanner.

tube. Third, the beam is collimated to pass through only the slice of interest. The beam is attenuated by the patient, and the detector then measures the transmitted photons. Fourth, the detectors convert the x-ray photons into an electrical signal (analog data), which is subsequently converted by the analog-to-digital converter (ADC) into digital data. Finally, the digital data is sent to the computer for image reconstruction.

Self-Assessment Questions will be based on each of the following Keywords and Concepts

- Slice-by-slice data acquisition
- Volume data acquisition

- Data acquisition beam geometries
- Pencil-beam geometry
- Fan-beam geometry
- CT scanner generations
- Multislice CT
- Spiral beam path (geometry)
- Helical beam path (geometry)
- Dual-Source CT Scanner
- Data acquisition components

Challenge Questions

Answer the following questions to check your understanding of the materials studied.

True (T)/False (F)

1. Data acquisition principles in CT include systematic methods of acquiring attenuation data from the patient.
2. The first step in producing CT images is image reconstruction.
3. The collection of attenuation data from the patient during CT scanning is referred to as *data acquisition*.
4. The current method of data acquisition in CT is volume CT, which implies that multiple slices are collected during a single revolution of the x-ray tube and detectors.
5. The method described in question 4 is referred to as *spiral/helical CT scanning*.
6. *Conventional CT* is a term used to describe the acquisition of one slice per revolution of the x-ray tube and detectors around the patient.
7. *Volume data acquisition* refers to the use of a spiral/helical beam geometry to scan the patient in an effort to obtain multiple slices per revolution of the x-ray tube and detectors.
8. Single-slice spiral/helical CT is characterized by the acquisition of a single slice during one revolution of the x-ray tube and detectors while the patient moves through the gantry aperture.
9. The beam geometry used in modern MSCT scanners use a pencil beam.
10. MSCT scanners with 64–320 slices per revolution use a cone-beam geometry.

11. The x-ray tube and detectors are among the major components for CT data acquisition.
12. X-ray beam filters (filtration) and x-ray beam-shaping collimators (collimation) are not CT data acquisition components.
13. The detector electronics are not part of the CT data acquisition components.

Multiple Choice

1. Which of the following are relevant to the data acquisition principles used by the CT scanner?
   1. Conventional single-slice CT
   2. Slice-by-slice acquisition per revolution of the x-ray tube and detectors
   3. Multislice acquisition per revolution of the x-ray tube and detectors
   4. Volume CT data acquisition
      A. 1 only
      B. 1 and 2
      C. 1, 2, and 3
      D. 1, 2, 3, and 4
2. The specific term used to describe the acquisition of multiple slices per revolution of the x-ray tube and detectors in CT is:
   A. Single-slice CT data acquisition
   B. Multi-slice CT image reconstruction
   C. Multi-slice CT data acquisition
   D. Multiple detector array acquisition
3. The continuous rotation of the x-ray tube and detectors in MSCT scanners is made possible by:
   A. Slip rings
   B. Two-dimensional detector array
   C. Special x-ray beam collimators
   D. A and C are correct.
4. The term used to describe the size, shape, motion, and path traced by the x-ray tube and detectors during CT scanning is:
   A. The x-ray beam geometry
   B. The x-ray beam collimation
   C. The category of CT scanner generation
   D. Spiral CT

5. Which of the following generations of CT scanners is based on the use of a single detector and in which the x-ray tube and detector rotate 180° using a pencil-beam geometry?
   A. First-generation scanners
   B. Second-generation scanners
   C. Third-generation scanners
   D. MSCT scanners

6. Which of the following generations of CT scanners is based on the use of a small array of detectors and in which the x-ray tube and detector rotate 180° using a small fan-beam geometry?
   A. First-generation scanners
   B. Second-generation scanners
   C. Third-generation scanners
   D. MSCT scanners

7. Which of the following generations of CT scanners is based on the use of a large array of detectors and in which the x-ray tube and detector rotate 360° using a wide fan-beam geometry?
   A. First-generation scanners
   B. Second-generation scanners
   C. Third-generation scanners
   D. MSCT scanners

8. The x-ray beam geometry that is used in MSCT scanners is:
   A. Pencil-beam geometry
   B. Small fan beam
   C. Wide fan beam
   D. A slit-beam geometry

9. The path traced by the x-ray beam as the patient moves through the gantry aperture in MSCT scanning describes a:
   A. Spiral
   B. Helix
   C. Straight line
   D. A and B are correct.

10. The scan time in CT is:
    A. Directly proportional to the number of detectors
    B. Related to the type of reconstruction algorithms used
    C. Directly proportional to the number of analog-to-digital converters
    D. Inversely proportional to the number of detectors

11. Which of the following is not a major component of the data acquisition system?
    A. X-ray tube
    B. Detectors
    C. Reconstruction algorithm
    D. X-ray beam filter and collimator

12. The data acquisition component that plays a major role in shaping the x-ray beam in CT scanning is the:
    A. Focal spot
    B. Filter
    C. Collimator
    D. Detector electronics

Short Answers

1. What are the two methods of acquiring attenuation data from the patient during CT scanning?
2. What is meant by the term *volume data acquisition*?
3. What is the major advantage of volume data acquisition?
4. Briefly describe the nature of the fan-beam geometry.
5. Explain the difference between second-generation and third-generation CT scanner beam geometries.
6. Describe the x-ray beam geometry of a spiral/helical CT scanner
7. What is the mathematical relationship between the number of detectors and scan time?
8. Identify the major components of the CT data acquisition system
9. State which system component is intended to shape the x-ray beam in CT.
10. Describe the key function of each of the major components of the data acquisition system.

Answers to Challenge Questions

True/False

1. T	6. F	11. T
2. F	7. T	12. F
3. T	8. F	13. F
4. F	9. F	
5. T	10. T	

Multiple Choice

1. D	5. A	9. D
2. C	6. B	10. D
3. A	7. C	11. C
4. A	8. C	12. B

Short Answer

1. The two methods of acquiring data from the patient during CT scanning are (i) slice-by-slice data acquisition and (ii) volume data acquisition. The former involves the following steps:
   A. The patient is positioned for the scan.
   B. The x-ray tube and detectors rotate around the patient for 360° and scan only one slice during this rotation.
   C. Scanning stops so that the patient can be positioned for the next slice.
   D. Scanning resumes.
   These steps are also called *stop-and-go*, and the data acquisition may also be called stop-and-go.
   This interscan delay led to the introduction of single-slice spiral/helical CT (SSCT), where only one slice is acquired per revolution (360°) of the tube and detectors. This method requires the use of a slip ring as part of the system components.

2. The second method of data collection in CT is volume data acquisition. This method requires the use of a slip ring on the scanner to allow the x-ray tube and detectors to rotate continuously as the patient moves simultaneously through the gantry aperture, to collect multiple slices per revolution of the tube and detectors (MSCT). The beam path traced by this method is referred to as a spiral or a helix, and hence the terms *spiral* CT scanning or *helical* CT scanning.

3. The major purpose of volume data acquisition or spiral/helical CT scanning is to increase the volume coverage speed performance compared to SSCT, where a one-dimensional detector array is used to acquire only one slice in spiral/helical mode. Volume coverage is increased since MSCT scanners use two-dimensional detector arrays to obtain multiple slices per revolution. State-of-the-art MSCT scanners are based on the use of 64–320 slices per revolution. This feature increases the volume coverage speed.

4. Since two-dimensional detector arrays are essential system components of MSCT scanners, the x-ray beam has to be opened to cover the area of these arrays; this creates a beam that resembles a fan, and hence the term *fan-beam geometry*. For MSCT scanners that use 320 detector elements, the beam has to be opened wider to cover the entire detector array. The beam geometry, in this case, is referred to as *cone-beam geometry*.

5. Two major differences between the second and third generations are as follows:

   A. Second-generation CT scanner beam geometry is based on rotating the x-ray beam and one-dimensional detector array 180° using a small fan-beam geometry. The tube and detectors first translate across the patient, followed by rotation and subsequent translation until the scanning occurs for 180°. This is referred to as a *translate/rotate beam geometry*.

   B. Third-generation CT scanner beam geometry is based on rotating the x-ray tube and one-dimensional detector array 360° using a wider fan-beam geometry. There is no translated motion.

6. Spiral/helical CT scanner beam geometries are based on the use of a wider fan beam to cover a two-dimensional detector array. The tube and detector array rotate continuously around the patient, who moves simultaneously through the scanner gantry. This continuous motion of the tube and detectors is made possible using slip rings.

7. The mathematical relationship between scan time and detectors is that the scan time is inversely proportional to the number of detectors. More detectors means shorter scan times.

8. The major components of the data acquisition system include:
   ○ The x-ray tube
   ○ The x-ray beam filter
   ○ The collimator
   ○ The object to be imaged (phantom or patient)
   ○ The detectors
   ○ The detector electronics (including the analog-to-digital converters)

9. The system component intended to shape the x-ray beam in CT is the filter. It is a specially designed filter to ensure that the beam reaching the detectors is uniform. This is important in order to use Beer-Lambert's law of attenuation so that the linear attenuation coefficient (μ) can be calculated.

10. The key function of each of the data acquisition systems is as follows:
    ○ The x-ray tube produces x-rays needed to image the patient.
    ○ The x-ray beam filter shapes and filters the x-ray beam to ensure a more uniform beam at the detectors.
    ○ The collimator shapes the beam to ensure that x-ray photons fall only upon the detectors.
    ○ The object to be imaged provides x-ray transmission data or attenuation data.
    ○ The detectors convert x-ray photons into electrical signals.
    ○ The detector electronics (including the analog-to-digital converters) convert electrical signals (analog data) into digital data for processing by a digital computer.

IDENTIFYING AREAS TO STUDY

A. Make a list of topics and/or questions that are still not clear to you after studying this chapter.
B. See the instructor for clarification and/or consolidation of the material.

3

X-Ray Tubes, Generators, Filtration, and Collimation in CT

PRIOR READING ASSIGNMENT

Before attempting to answer these review questions, read the following brief summary notes on this topic.

This chapter will review the essential features of x-ray tubes and generators used in CT, as well as filtration and collimation schemes. Specifically, the generator provides the x-ray tube with the high voltage needed to produce x-rays. CT generators are high-frequency generators. X-ray tubes used in CT are rotating anode tubes with compound anode disks. These tubes have high heat loading capacity and very fast heat dissipation rates.

The filter used in CT is specially designed to ensure that the beam reaching the detectors is uniform. The fundamental filtration scheme used in CT is shown in Figure 3.1.

Computed Tomography: Physics and Technology A Self Assessment Guide,
Second Edition. Euclid Seeram.
© 2022 John Wiley & Sons Ltd. Published 2022 by John Wiley & Sons Ltd.

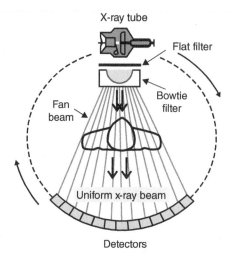

Figure 3.1 **The major elements of x-ray beam filtration used in CT.**

Collimation is an important system component in CT. The basic collimation approach is illustrated in Figure 3.2 and includes, in particular, pre-patient and pre-detector collimators. Slice thickness is

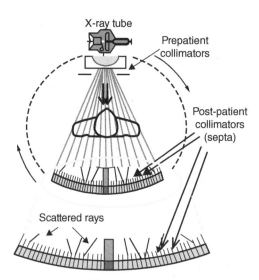

Figure 3.2 **The basic components of the collimation approach used in a CT scanner.**

also defined by the collimator. A key design of the collimator used in multislice CT (MSCT) scanners is what is referred to as *adaptive* or *dynamic* collimation.

Self-Assessment Questions will be based on each of the following Keywords and Concepts

- X-ray generator
- High-frequency generator
- Stationary x-ray tube
- Rotating anode x-ray tube
- Thermionic emission
- Potential difference
- Anode disk
- Focal spot
- Heat storage capacity
- Heat units
- Filtration
- Bowtie filter
- Collimation
- Adaptive or dynamic collimation

Challenge Questions

Answer the following questions to check your understanding of the materials studied.

True (T)/False (F)

1. The purpose of the x-ray generator is to provide low voltage to the x-ray tube.
2. The x-ray generator changes the low-voltage, low-frequency AC waveform to supply the x-ray tube with high-voltage, high-frequency direct current of almost constant potential.
3. High-frequency generators are used in CT.
4. The voltage ripple from a high-frequency generator is less than 1%, compared with 4% from a 3-phase, 12-pulse generator.
5. The number of x-ray photons coming from the x-ray tube is determined by the milliamperes (mA).
6. The quality of the photons from the x-ray tube is determined by the kilovolts (kV) applied to the tube.

7. Modern-day CT scanners use rotating anode x-ray tubes with anode disks made of two or more materials.
8. Electrons emitted from the filament of the x-ray tube are the result of thermionic emission.
9. The x-ray tube current is the current (amperes) applied to the filament of the tube.
10. The heat storage capacity of the x-ray tube is expressed in heat units (HUs).
11. The CT filter does not affect the "hardness" of the x-ray beam.
12. The filter in CT is specially designed ("bowtie") to protect the patient from unnecessary radiation.
13. The collimator section at the distal end of the collimator assembly plays a role in defining the thickness of the section to be imaged in CT.
14. Adaptive collimation in MSCT scanners is intended to eliminate the effects of overranging and overbeaming.

Multiple Choice

1. The purpose of the x-ray generator in CT is to:
   A. Provide low voltage to the x-ray tube
   B. Provide high-voltage alternating current (AC) to the x-ray tube
   C. Provide high-voltage direct current (DC) to the x-ray tube
   D. Ensure that the x-ray tube produces a homogeneous beam of radiation
2. Which type of x-ray generator is used in CT?
   A. High-frequency x-ray generator
   B. Single-phase x-ray generator
   C. Six-pulse, three-phase x-ray generator
   D. Twelve-pulse, three-phase x-ray generator
3. The x-ray generator with the highest percentage ripple (less than 1%) is the:
   A. Twelve-pulse, three-phase generator
   B. Six-pulse, three-phase generator
   C. High-frequency generator
   D. Single-phase generator
4. CT scanners operate with rotating-anode diagnostic x-ray tubes because they:
   A. Provide high radiation intensities needed for high-contrast images
   B. Have offset filaments compared with stationary-anode tubes

C. Conduct heat faster than stationary-anode tubes
D. Rotate with the detectors as the patient moves simultaneously through the gantry aperture
5. The radiation beam emanating from the x-ray tube used in MSCT scanners is:
   A. Homogeneous
   B. Heterogeneous
   C. Monochromatic
   D. A low-intensity beam where all photons have the same energy
6. Which of the following is responsible for accelerating the electrons from the filament to the anode target?
   A. mA
   B. kV
   C. Filament current in amperes
   D. Anode rotation speed
7. What is the source of x-rays in the function of the x-ray tube?
   A. The filament
   B. The focusing cup of the cathode
   C. The target of the anode disk
   D. The x-ray generator
8. Rotating anode disks have been redesigned to accommodate more heat storage capacity and faster heat dissipation rates. Heat storage capacity is expressed in:
   A. Hounsfield units
   B. Heat units
   C. Gigabytes per mAs applied to the tube
   D. Exposure units
9. The purpose of the x-ray tube envelope is to:
   1. Ensure that a vacuum is maintained
   2. Provide structural support for the anode
   3. Provide high-voltage insulation between the anode and cathode
   4. Provide structural support for all cathode components
      A. 1 only
      B. 1 and 2
      C. 1, 2, and 4
      D. All are correct
10. Which of the following x-ray tube designs has more heat storage capacity and faster heat dissipation rates?
    A. Rotating anode with a tungsten target
    B. Stationary anode with a rhenium target

C. Rotating anode with a rhenium-tungsten (RH) target

D. Rotating anode with a rhenium-tungsten-molybdenum (RTM) target

11. X-ray tubes used in present-day MSCT scanners have:

A. Completely glass envelopes

B. Glass-metal envelopes

C. Completely metal envelopes

D. Complete ceramic envelopes

12. Which component of a CT scanner is designed to shape the energy distribution across the radiation beam to produce a more uniform beam at the CT detectors?

A. The target of the anode disk

B. The pre-patient collimators

C. The bowtie filter

D. The pre-detector collimator

13. The major purpose of pre-patient collimation is to:

A. Ensure a constant beam width at the detector

B. Provide a constant beam energy at the detector

C. Define the degree of radiation protection to the patient

D. Eliminate scattered radiation at the detectors

14. The purpose of adaptive or dynamic collimation in MSCT scanners is to:

A. Reduce any scattered radiation reaching the detectors

B. Eliminate overbeaming effects

C. Eliminate overranging effects

D. Both B and C are correct.

Short Answers

1. What is the purpose of an x-ray generator in a CT imaging system?

2. What type of generator is used in current MSCT scanners? State the percentage ripple of this generator.

3. What are the key characteristics of a high-frequency generator used in any x-ray imaging modality?

4. Describe the essential technical components of a rotating-anode x-ray tube used in CT.

5. What is meant by the acronym RTM? State the reason for its use in an x-ray tube.

6. What is the purpose of a filter in diagnostic radiography?

7. Explain the nature of filtration in CT.

8. Describe the major components of collimation in CT.

9. What is an adaptive or dynamic collimator?
10. State the difference between the terms *overbeaming* and *overranging* as used in MSCT scanners.

Answers to Challenge Questions

True/False

1. F	6. T	11. T
2. T	7. T	12. F
3. T	8. T	13. T
4. T	9. F	14. T
5. T	10. T	

Multiple Choice

1. C	6. B	11. C
2. A	7. C	12. C
3. C	8. B	13. A
4. A	9. D	14. D
5. B	10. D	

Short Answer

1. The major purpose of the x-ray generator in the CT imaging system is to provide the x-ray tube with a high voltage of the correct frequency and current needed to produce x-rays, especially in MSCT scanners.
2. The current state-of-the-art generator used in CT is a high-frequency generator with a ripple of less than 1%, compared with 4% from a 3-phase, 12-pulse generator. This makes the high-frequency generator more efficient at x-ray production than its predecessor.
3. This is a special generator consisting of many electrical components, which serve to:
   A. Convert the low-frequency (60 Hz), low-voltage alternating current (AC) from the electrical power coming into the hospital to high-frequency (about 150 Hz), high-voltage (DC) direct current.
   B. This conversion is accomplished by the use of rectifiers, capacitors, inverter circuits, high-voltage transformers, and

high-voltage capacitors (see Figure 5.2 in *CT at a Glance* [Seeram 2018]) to produce x-rays efficiently with a ripple of less than 1%.

4. The major technical components of a rotating anode x-ray tube for use in CT are:

   ○ A cathode assembly and an anode, both encased in a tube envelope that ensures a vacuum.

   ○ The cathode assembly consists of a filament made of a thin tungsten wire wound in a helical fashion. The filament is positioned in a focusing cup, is heated by a current (filament current) passing through it, and emits electrons through a process referred to as *thermionic emission*. The electrons are then accelerated to strike the anode. The flow of electrons across the tube is called the *tube current* or mA.

   ○ There is a potential difference (kV) between the cathode and anode to accelerate the electrons to strike the target of the anode.

   ○ The anode is a rotating anode and consists of a certain defined region that the electrons strike to produce x-rays. This is the x-ray tube target, consisting of an active region called the *focal spot*.

   ○ The production of x-rays causes the anode disk to heat up. The amount of heat can be expressed by what is referred to as a *heat unit* (HU). When 1 mA, 1 kV is applied to the tube for 1 second, the amount of HU produced is 1. The heat storage capacity of the tube is expressed as HUs. Fast heat dissipation rates are essential to CT imaging.

   ○ The tube envelope ensures a vacuum, provides structural support for the anode and cathode structures, and provides high-voltage insulation between the anode and cathode. Today, tubes with metal envelopes are not common since they can accommodate the use of larger anode disks and have higher heat storage capacities than their previous counterparts.

5. Early disks were made of pure tungsten, but because of the limitations in heat storage capacity, materials such as RTM and other combinations of alloys are now popular. Disks with two or more materials used in their design are called *compound anode disks*.

6. The major purpose of filtration in diagnostic radiography is to protect the patient by removing low-energy photons from the beam. These photons are absorbed by the patient since they do

not have enough energy to penetrate the patient. Since low-energy photons are removed, the beam becomes "harder" or more penetrating. The average energy of the beam is increased.

7. The filtration scheme is illustrated in Figure 3.1, which shows the position of the filters in a CT imaging system. Two types of filters are shown: a flat filter and a bowtie filter. Since the x-ray beam from the tube is heterogeneous (consisting of high- and low-energy photons), the design of the filters serves two major purposes:

A. The flat filter removes low-energy photons since they do not have enough energy to reach the detectors. They are absorbed by the patient and therefore result in unnecessary doses to the patient. The beam then becomes "harder" (more penetrating) and leads to what are referred to as *beam hardening artifacts*.

B. On the other hand, the bowtie filter shapes the beam to provide a more uniform beam at the detectors so that Beer-Lambert's law of attenuation can be used in CT to calculate the linear attenuation coefficients (μs) of the tissues traversed by the radiation beam. This is the mathematical problem in CT.

8. Figure 3.2 illustrates the collimation scheme used in CT scanners. There are adjustable pre-patient collimators, post-patient collimators, and pre-detector collimators. The collimators at the x-ray tube and those close to the detectors are perfectly aligned to ensure a constant beam at the detector. The collimators positioned close to the detectors also shape the beam and remove scattered radiation in an effort to improve image quality. The collimator section at the distal end of the collimator assembly also helps define the thickness of the slice to be imaged. Various slice thicknesses are available depending on the type of scanner.

9. MSCT scanners now use *adaptive collimation schemes* to address the problems of overranging and overbeaming by adjusting the collimators at the start and end of the scan. In this way, portions of the beam to which the patient is exposed are blocked in the z-direction.

10. As noted in the answer to question 9, overbeaming and overranging are eliminated using adaptive collimation. While overbeaming means that the beam is somewhat wider than the detector, overranging means that the patient is exposed to radiation beyond the needed length of the scan (at the beginning and end of the scan).

Subsequently, these effects increase the dose to the patient. For example, overranging can result in an increase in the dose from 5 to 30%.

IDENTIFYING AREAS TO STUDY

A. Make a list of topics and/or questions that are still not clear to you after studying this chapter.

B. See the instructor for clarification and/or consolidation of the material.

4

Radiation Attenuation in CT: Essential Physics

PRIOR READING ASSIGNMENT

Before attempting to answer these review questions, read the following brief summary notes on this topic.

This chapter reviews the fundamental elements of the attenuation of radiation as it passes through the patient. While 100% of photons fall upon the surface of the patient, only about 3% reach the detectors. *Attenuation* is the reduction of the beam intensity as it passes through an object such as the patient. Additionally, attenuation of homogeneous and heterogeneous beams is described, followed by an overview of Beer-Lambert's law, which is an important topic in CT physics.

Attenuation measurements are used in CT to produce what is referred to as *CT numbers*, which are digital images (numbers) of the patient's sectional anatomy. These numbers are referred to as *integers*. An integer can be a positive number, a negative number, or

Computed Tomography: Physics and Technology A Self Assessment Guide,
Second Edition. Euclid Seeram.
© 2022 John Wiley & Sons Ltd. Published 2022 by John Wiley & Sons Ltd.

a zero. These numbers must be converted into a grayscale image in which higher numbers represent white and lower numbers represent black, with shades of gray in between. The gray scale can be manipulated by a technique called *windowing* to display shades of gray that the observer can see. Finally, all tissues are assigned CT numbers. For example, while bone has a range of CT numbers from 800 to 3000, muscle has a range of CT numbers from 35 to 50. The CT numbers for water, fat, and air are 0, −100, and −1000, respectively.

Self-Assessment Questions will be based on each of the following Keywords and Concepts

- Radiation attenuation
- Factors affecting attenuation
- Homogeneous beam
- Heterogeneous beam
- Relative transmission value
- Attenuation of a homogeneous beam
- Attenuation of a heterogeneous beam
- Beam hardening
- Beer-Lambert's law
- CT numbers
- CT numbers and the gray scale
- Windowing
- CT numbers for various tissues

Challenge Questions

Answer the following questions to check your understanding of the materials studied.

True (T)/False (F)

1. Attenuation is the removal of low-energy photons from the x-ray beam.
2. Attenuation refers to the reduction of the intensity of the beam as it passes through the patient.
3. About 3% of the beam falls upon the detector after it (the beam) has passed through the patient.

4. Attenuation depends only on the atomic number of the tissue that the beam passes through.
5. The effective atomic density (atoms/volume) affects attenuation.
6. The relative transmission values or attenuation measurements are directly proportional to the intensity of x-rays at the detector.
7. The attenuation value is a ratio of the intensity of x-rays at the x-ray tube to the intensity of x-rays at the detector.
8. During attenuation of the photons for a homogeneous beam, equal thicknesses of materials remove equal amounts of radiation.
9. During attenuation of the x-ray beam for a heterogeneous beam, the beam becomes harder; that is, the average energy of the beam increases.
10. Beer-Lambert's law only holds true for a heterogeneous beam of radiation.
11. CT numbers are integers calculated from the attenuation of the tissues relative to water.
12. CT numbers for a slice of tissue must be converted to a grayscale image for viewing and interpretation.
13. A CT grayscale image can be manipulated by a digital image processing procedure called *windowing*.
14. The CT number for water is −100.
15. The CT number for air is −1000.
16. CT numbers for bone may vary between 800 and 3000.

Multiple Choice

1. Attenuation is defined as:
   A. The calculation of CT numbers
   B. The production of scattered radiation
   C. A decrease in the intensity of x-rays as they pass through an object (patient)
   D. An increase in the intensity of x-rays as they pass through an object
2. The fractional reduction of the intensity of a beam of radiation per unit thickness of the medium traversed is defined as:
   A. An integer referred to as a CT number
   B. The linear attenuation coefficient (μ)
   C. The base of the natural logarithm
   D. The log of the ratio of the source intensity to the intensity at the detector

3. Radiation attenuation in CT depends on:
   A. Density of the absorber
   B. Atomic number of the absorber
   C. Energy of the radiation beam
   D. All are correct.

4. The unit of the linear attenuation coefficient (μ) is:
   A. gm/cm
   B. cm^2
   C. mm^{-1}
   D. cm^{-1}

5. Using this diagram, where
      I_0 = Intensity of radiation from the x-ray tube
      I = Intensity of radiation at the CT detector
      μ = Attenuation coefficient
      x = Thickness of the tissue
   the correct equation describing Beer-Lambert's law of exponential attenuation is:
   A. $I = I_0 e^{-\mu \Delta x}$
   B. $I = I_0 e^{\mu \Delta x}$
   C. $I_0 = I e^{-\mu \Delta x}$
   D. $I/I = e^{-\mu \Delta x}$

6. In the attenuation of a homogeneous beam of radiation:
   A. Radiation is not attenuated exponentially.
   B. A greater fraction of the low-energy photons remains.
   C. There is a change in the number of photons.
   D. The beam becomes more penetrating (harder).

7. For the attenuation of a heterogeneous beam of radiation:
   A. The exponential law holds true.
   B. A greater fraction of the low-energy photons remains.
   C. There is a change in the beam quantity and no change in beam quality.
   D. The beam becomes more penetrating (harder).

8. Which of the following increases radiation attenuation?
   A. Decreasing the density of the absorber
   B. Decreasing the atomic number of the absorber
   C. Increasing the radiation energy
   D. Decreasing the radiation energy

9. The CT number is:
    A. A number calculated for each voxel (volume element) in the slice of tissue to be imaged based on the attenuation coefficients of the tissues within the voxel
    B. A number that denotes how many attenuation coefficients are in the tissue voxel
    C. A number indicating how many electrons are in the tissue voxel
    D. A number used by the pioneer Hounsfield to describe the degree of radiation transmission through the patient

10. Which of the following is not used to calculate CT numbers?
    A. Attenuation coefficient of the tissue
    B. Attenuation coefficient of water
    C. The thickness of the slice being imaged
    D. Manufacturer's scaling or contrast factor

11. Which of the following algebraic expressions is used to calculate CT numbers, where the attenuation coefficients for tissue is μ_t and the attenuation coefficient for water is μ_w? The manufacturer's contrast factor is K.
    A. $CT = \mu_{w-}\mu_t/\mu_w \times K$
    B. $CT = \mu_{t-}\mu_w/\mu_w\ K$
    C. $CT = \mu_{t-}\mu_w/\mu_{w\ x}\ K$
    D. $CT = \mu_{w+}\mu_{t\ x}\ K$

12. The CT number is also referred to as the:
    A. Euclid unit (EU)
    B. Roentgen unit (RU)
    C. Cormack unit (CU)
    D. Hounsfield unit (HU)

13. Given that the μ for bone is 0.380, the μ for water is 0.190, and the scaling factor for the scanner is 1000, the CT number for bone is:
    A. +1000
    B. −1000
    C. +380
    D. −190

14. Which of the following affects the value of the CT number?
    A. The scan motion of the x-ray tube and detectors
    B. The number of detectors
    C. The number of slices imaged per volume of tissue
    D. The energy of the radiation beam

15. Arrange the following numbered list in decreasing order of CT numbers: 1 = bone; 2 = air; 3 = water; 4 = muscle; and 5 = fat:
    A. 1, 2, 4, 5, 3
    B. 1, 4, 3, 5, 2
    C. 1, 5, 3, 2, 4
    D. 1, 3, 4, 5, 2

16. The purpose of windowing the CT image is to:
    A. Change the numerical image to a grayscale image
    B. Manipulate the gray scale to produce a grayscale CT image
    C. Assign the CT number +1000 a shade of white
    D. Assign the CT number −1000 a shade of black

17. What is the approximate range of CT numbers for muscle?
    A. 100–200
    B. 0–100
    C. 35–50
    D. 0–35

18. What is the CT number for fat?
    A. −100
    B. −1000
    C. 0
    D. 100

Short Answers

1. What is radiation attenuation, and why is it important to CT?
2. Explain the fundamental difference between a homogeneous and a heterogeneous beam of radiation.
3. Write out the algebraic expression for the relative transmission measurement.
4. Briefly explain the attenuation of a homogeneous beam of radiation.
5. Briefly explain the attenuation of a heterogeneous beam of radiation.
6. Write out the algebraic expression for Beer-Lambert's law, and state why it is important in CT.
7. Explain briefly what is meant by a CT number, and write out the algebraic expression used to calculate a CT number.
8. Show the calculation of the CT number for water.
9. What are gray levels, and how are they converted to a gray scale?
10. Write out the CT number range for bone and muscle, and list the CT numbers for water, fat, and air.

Answers to Challenge Questions

True/False

1. F	7. T	13. T
2. T	8. T	14. F
3. T	9. T	15. T
4. F	10. F	16. T
5. T	11. T	
6. F	12. T	

Multiple Choice

1. C	7. D	13. A
2. B	8. D	14. D
3. D	9. A	15. D
4. D	10. C	16. B
5. A	11. C	17. C
6. C	12. D	18. A

Short Answer

1. Radiation attenuation is the reduction of the beam intensity as it passes through an object (patient). Attenuation is important in CT because mathematics is used to calculate the linear attenuation coefficients (μs) for all tissues being imaged. μ is defined as the fractional reduction of the radiation beam as it passes through tissues, and it is used to calculate CT numbers, which are subsequently converted into a grayscale image (a CT image)
2. Two types of radiation beams are a homogeneous beam and a heterogeneous beam. In a homogeneous beam, all photons have the same energy. In a heterogeneous beam, photons have different energies.
3. The algebraic expression is:

$$\text{Relative transmission} = \text{Log} \frac{\text{Intensity of x-rays at the source } (I_0)}{\text{Intensity of x-rays at the detector } (I)}$$

4. The attenuation of a homogeneous beam of radiation is important in CT since this attenuation describes Beer-Lambert's law of exponential attenuation. There are three important characteristics to note when a homogeneous beam travels through water:

A. If 1000 photons enter a block of water, due to attenuation, 32 photons exit the water block. This is a reduction in the intensity of the beam (attenuation). In particular, the number of photons is reduced.

B. The initial beam energy (beam quality) has not changed. Photons enter the water block at 40 kV and exit the block with the same 40 kV energy.

C. Equal thicknesses of blocks of water remove the same number of photons from the beam.

5. A heterogeneous beam consists of photons with different energies, and these photons have low and high energies. While high-energy photons penetrate the patient and reach the detector to create the image, low-energy photons are essentially absorbed by the patient. Four noteworthy points are:

A. Attenuation is not exponential, and therefore both the number of photons (intensity) and the quality (energy) of the photons change.

B. If 1000 photons enter a block of water at 40 kV energy, 32 photons exit with a mean energy of 52 kV.

C. Equal thicknesses of blocks of water do not remove the same number of photons.

D. Since lower-energy photons are absorbed, the mean energy of the beam increases (point B), and therefore the beam becomes more penetrating (harder).

6. Beer-Lambert's law is expressed as follows:

$$I = I_0 e^{-\mu \Delta x}$$

It is important in CT because it is used to calculate the attenuation coefficients (μs) of the various tissues traversed by the radiation beam as the patient is being scanned.

7. A CT number is an integer (0, positive number, or negative number) calculated from attenuation measurements (values) obtained from the patient during the data collection. A CT image is made up of a number of integers that represents a digital CT image. The CT number is calculated from the attenuation measurements using this formula

$$CT\,number = \frac{\mu_{tissue} - \mu_{water}}{\mu_{water}} \cdot K$$

where μ_{tissue} is the attenuation coefficient of the measured tissue, μ_{water} is the attenuation coefficient of water, and K is a constant. The value of K determines the contrast factor or scaling factor.

8. The CT number for water = $\mu_{water-}\mu_{water/}\mu_{water}$. K

9. In digital image processing, gray levels are numerical values that create a matrix of numbers (CT numbers) that can be displayed for viewing. However, radiologists prefer to view and interpret grayscale images on a monitor. Therefore, the numerical values from the digital image must be converted into grayscale images displayed on a monitor, such that the higher numbers are white and the lower numbers are dark. Numbers between the higher and lower numbers are shaded gray. See Figure 8.2 in *CT at a Glance* (Seeram 2018).

10. Generally, bone has a range of CT numbers from 800 to 3000, while muscle has a range of CT numbers from 35 to 50. The CT numbers for water, fat, and air are 0, −100, and −1000, respectively.

IDENTIFYING AREAS TO STUDY

A. Make a list of topics and/or questions that are still not clear to you after studying this chapter.

B. See the instructor for clarification and/or consolidation of the material.

5

CT Detector Technology: Fundamentals

PRIOR READING ASSIGNMENT

Before attempting to answer these review questions, read the following brief summary notes on this topic.

These review notes discuss several topics such as the location and purpose of detectors in CT, essential characteristics of detectors, types of detectors and their function, and the data acquisition system (DAS).

CT detectors are located opposite the x-ray tube, are in perfect alignment with the tube, and are coupled to the *detector electronics*, which essentially consist of the analog-to-digital converters (ADCs). CT detectors have a two-fold function: to capture the transmitted x-rays from the patient and convert the transmitted photons into digital data using ADCs.

Computed Tomography: Physics and Technology A Self Assessment Guide,
Second Edition. Euclid Seeram.
© 2022 John Wiley & Sons Ltd. Published 2022 by John Wiley & Sons Ltd.

Major characteristics of CT detectors include efficiency, stability, response time, dynamic range, and afterglow. While *efficiency* refers to the ability to capture, absorb, and convert x-ray photons to electrical signals, *stability* is the steadiness of the detector response. If the system is not stable, frequent calibrations are required to render the signals useful. Additionally, the *response time* of the detector refers to the speed with which the detector can detect an x-ray event and recover to detect another event.

There are three types of detectors: energy-integrating (EI) detectors (conventional CT detectors, the more common CT detectors), dual-layer detectors, and direct conversion detectors. EI detectors use a scintillation crystal to convert x-ray photons into light photons and photodiodes to convert light into electrical signals, which are then digitized and sent to the CT computer for image reconstruction. Scintillation crystals such as sodium iodide, calcium fluoride, and bismuth germinate were used in the past; however, cadmium tungstate and rare earth oxides such as yttria and gadolinium oxysulfide (GOS) ultrafast ceramic (UFC) are used today. More recently, lutetium (Lu)-based garnet has been introduced for use in CT. Dual-layer detector technology is made up of two layers of scintillators: a top layer of a low-density scintillator (ZnSe), which absorbs low-energy x-ray photons that are subsequently converted to light photons, and a bottom layer of a high-density scintillator (GOS), which absorbs high-energy x-ray photons that are subsequently converted to light photons. An important component of CT detectors is an application-specific integrated circuit (ASIC) designed for ADC and integration of the two energies.

In 2021, the Food and Drug Administration (FDA) approved the use of photocounting detectors that use, for example, cadmium telluride (semiconductor) for clinical CT use.

The DAS (detector electronics) measures transmitted radiation, codes these measurements into binary data, and finally transmits binary data to the digital computer.

Self-Assessment Questions will be based on each of the following Keywords and Concepts

- Location of the detectors
- Purpose of the detectors
- Efficiency of the detectors
- Stability of the detectors

- Response time of the detectors
- Dynamic range of the detectors
- Energy-integrating detector
- Dual-layer detector
- Direct conversion detector
- Scintillation crystals
- Low-density scintillator
- High-density scintillator
- DAS

Challenge Questions

Answer the following questions to check your understanding of the materials studied.

True (T)/False (F)

1. CT detectors are located just below the patient table.
2. CT detectors are always coupled to the unit containing the detector electronics.
3. ADCs are major technical components of the detector electronics.
4. One purpose of the CT detector array is to capture scattered x-rays from the patient to create the image.
5. CT detectors convert x-ray photons to electrical signals, which must be digitized and sent to a computer for processing.
6. The response time of a CT detector is not one of the key characteristics of detectors used in CT.
7. The ratio of the largest signal to be measured to the precision of the smallest signal to be discriminated is referred to as the *dynamic range* of the detector.
8. *Afterglow* refers to the persistence of the image even after the radiation has been turned off. CT detectors should have low afterglow values.
9. The most common CT detector is the direct conversion detector, also referred to as a *photocounting detector* (PDC).
10. Scintillation energy-integrating detectors are commonly used in CT.
11. A high-density scintillator such as GOS is used in a dual-layer CT detector.
12. The detector electronics are also referred to as the DAS.

Multiple Choice

1. The CT detector is located:
   A. Above the patient table
   B. Under the patient table
   C. Before the ADCs
   D. In the CT gantry aperture where the patient is positioned

2. CT detectors capture photons transmitted through the patient, and these photons are subsequently converted into:
   A. An image
   B. Digital data
   C. Electrical signals
   D. Data for processing by a computer

3. Which of the following characteristics of CT detectors refers to the ability to capture, absorb, and convert x-ray photons to electrical signals?
   A. Response time
   B. Dynamic range
   C. Efficiency
   D. Stability

4. The steadiness of the CT detector response is referred to as:
   A. Stability
   B. Efficiency
   C. Dynamic range
   D. Response time

5. The ratio of the largest signal to be measured by the CT detector to the precision of the smallest signal to be discriminated is defined as the:
   A. Stability
   B. Efficiency
   C. Dynamic range
   D. Response time

6. For CT detectors, the persistence of the image even after the radiation has been turned off is referred to as:
   A. Stability
   B. Efficiency
   C. Dynamic range
   D. Afterglow

7. The most common of CT detectors is the:
   A. Energy-integrating detector
   B. Dual-layer detector

    C. Direct conversion detector

    D. Photon counting detector

8. The typical dynamic range of most CT scanners is about:

    A. 1 000 000 : 1

    B. 10 000 : 1

    C. 1000 : 1

    D. 100 : 1

9. Which of the following has not been used as a detector crystal in CT?

    A. Sodium iodide

    B. Calcium tungstate

    C. Bismuth germanate

    D. Cadmium tungstate

10. The signal from a CT detector goes directly to the:

    A. Computer

    B. Array processor

    C. Analog-to-digital converters

    D. Optical disk for storage

11. Which component of the DAS converts light photons to electrical signals?

    A. ADC

    B. Scintillation crystal

    C. ASIC

    D. Photodiode

12. Which component in CT detector technology is common to all three major types of CT detectors?

    A. AISC

    B. Sodium iodide

    C. Photodiode

    D. Ultrafast ceramic

13. Both low-density and high-density scintillators are common to:

    A. AISC

    B. Dual-layer detector

    C. Photon counting detector (direct conversion detector)

    D. Energy-integrating detector

14. The purpose of the data acquisition system in CT is:

    A. Measure transmitted radiation through the patient

    B. Encode transmission data into binary code

    C. Transmit binary code to a digital computer

    D. All of the above are correct.

Short Answers

1. What is the purpose of the detectors in a CT scanner?
2. Explain the flow of transmission data from the patient to the CT computer.
3. List five key characteristics of CT detectors, and state the meaning of each of them.
4. Describe the energy-integrating CT detector.
5. Describe the dual-layer CT detector.
6. Explain how a direct conversion CT detector works.
7. Describe the data acquisition system in CT.

Answers to Challenge Questions

True/False

1. T	5. T	9. F
2. T	6. F	10. T
3. T	7. T	11. T
4. F	8. T	12. T

Multiple Choice

1. B	6. D	11. D
2. C	7. A	12. A
3. C	8. A	13. B
4. A	9. B	14. D
5. C	10. C	

Short Answer

1. The purpose of the detectors in CT is two-fold:
   A. To capture the radiation transmitted through the patient
   B. To convert the x-ray photons into light, which is subsequently converted into electrical signals
2. The flow of transmission data from the patient to the CT computer consists of the following steps:
   A. The transmission radiation from the patient falls upon the detector.
   B. These x-ray photons are converted into light photons by the scintillation crystal in the detector.

C. The light photons are subsequently converted into electrical signals (analog signals) by the photodiodes.

D. These electrical signals are then converted to digital data by the ADCs.

E. The resulting digital data is sent to the computer for processing and image creation.

3. Five key characteristics of CT detectors include efficiency, stability, response time, dynamic range, and afterglow. While *efficiency* refers to the ability of the detector to capture, absorb, and convert x-ray photons into electrical signals, *stability* refers to the steadiness of the detector response. Furthermore, *response time* refers to the speed with which the detector can detect an x-ray event and recover to detect another event. The *dynamic range*, on the other hand, refers to the ratio of the largest signal to be measured by the CT detector to the precision of the smallest signal to be discriminated. This is about $1\,000\,000:1$ for CT scanners. Finally, *afterglow* refers to the persistence of the image even after the radiation has been turned off.

4. The basic functions of the energy-integrating CT detector are as follows:

A. X-ray photons from the patient fall upon the scintillation crystal of the detector.

B. The crystal converts x-ray photons into light photons

C. The light photons are then converted into electrical signals (analog signals) by the photo diode.

D. Associated electronics such as the ADCs convert the electrical signals into digital data.

E. The digital data are subsequently sent to the computer for processing and image creation.

5. Essentially, a dual-layer CT detector works as follows:

A. X-ray photons fall upon the scintillation crystals.

B. There are two layers of scintillation crystals: a top layer and a bottom layer.

C. While the top layer is made of a low-density scintillator such as zinc selenide (ZnSe), the bottom layer is made up of a high-density scintillator such as GOS.

D. ZnSe absorbs low-energy x-ray photons that are subsequently converted to light photons.

E. GOS, on the other hand, absorbs high-energy x-ray photons that are subsequently converted to light photons.

   F. Both top and bottom scintillators are coupled to a vertically positioned thin front-illuminated photodiode (FIP), which converts light into electrical signals.

   G. The FIP is placed under the scattered radiation grid so it will not compromise the detector's geometric efficiency.

   H. An ASIC is designed for analog-to-digital conversion and integration of the two energies: low- and high-energy spectra.

6. EI detectors are *indirect conversion detectors*; that is, x-ray photons are first converted to light, and then light photons are converted into electrical signals, which are subsequently digitized and fed into the computer for processing. The *direct conversion detector* is referred to as a PCD. The following is noteworthy:

   A. X-ray photons fall upon the *direct conversion material*. These materials are made of semiconductors that convert x-ray photons directly into electrical signals.

   B. Common semiconductors used in the construction of PCDs are cadmium telluride and cadmium zinc telluride; however, materials such as silicon and gallium arsenide have also been used.

   C. PCDs count the number of individual photons and carry energy information.

   D. As noted by Leng et al., "The output signal from a PCD is processed by multiple electronic comparators and counters, where the number of comparators and counters depends on the electronic design of the PCD and its ASICs. Each detected signal is compared with a voltage that has been calibrated to reflect a specified photon energy level, referred to as an energy threshold. When the energy level of a detected photon exceeds an energy threshold associated with a counter, the photon count is increased by one. In this manner, the number of photons that have energy equal to or greater than a specified energy level is measured. This process is enabled by the very fast ASIC, a key element in PCDs" (Leng et al. 2019).

   E. Leng et al. also state that "Photon-counting detector (PCD) CT is an emerging technology that has shown tremendous progress in the last decade. Various types of PCD CT systems have been developed to investigate the benefits of this technology, which include reduced electronic noise, increased contrast-to-noise ratio with iodinated contrast material and radiation dose efficiency, reduced beam-hardening and metal artifacts, extremely high spatial resolution (33 line pairs per centimeter), simultaneous multienergy data acquisition, and the ability to image with and differentiate among multiple CT contrast agents. PCD technology is described and compared with conventional CT detector technology. With the use of a whole-body research PCD CT system as an example, PCD technology and its use for in vivo high-spatial-resolution multienergy CT imaging is discussed. The potential clinical applications, diagnostic benefits, and challenges associated with this technology are then discussed, and examples with phantom, animal, and patient studies are provided" (Leng et al. 2019).

IDENTIFYING AREAS TO STUDY

A. Make a list of topics and/or questions that are still not clear to you after studying this chapter.
B. See the instructor for clarification and/or consolidation of the material.

6

Image Reconstruction in CT: Basic Principles

PRIOR READING ASSIGNMENT

Before attempting to answer these review questions, read the following brief summary notes:

1. Image reconstruction is the second of the three steps in the production of CT images.
2. Image reconstruction uses mathematics to reconstruct images of the patient's anatomy. In particular, algorithms are used to solve the sum of the attenuation coefficients (line integrals) collected by the data acquisition system, in which the x-ray tube and detectors rotate around the patient to collect x-ray transmission measurements (attenuation values) at various known locations.

Computed Tomography: Physics and Technology A Self Assessment Guide, Second Edition. Euclid Seeram.
© 2022 John Wiley & Sons Ltd. Published 2022 by John Wiley & Sons Ltd.

3. These algorithms fall into two categories: analytical methods and iterative methods.
4. Iterative algorithms are popular methods used in CT image reconstruction today.
5. Iterative methods have been developed for use in low-dose CT in an effort to reduce the dose to the patient.
6. More recently, artificial intelligence (AI) algorithms are used in low-dose CT imaging.
7. Deep learning (DL), a subset of machine learning (ML) algorithms, is now used in CT image reconstruction.

The use of AI in CT image reconstruction (see references)

Points 6 and 7 in the previous list introduce the use of AI in CT image reconstruction. This section describes AI and how DL algorithms are currently used in CT image reconstruction.

Iterative reconstruction algorithms are problematic due to long reconstruction times and specific features of noise that affect the appearance of images, especially with low-dose CT (LD-CT) techniques. For example, it has been reported that images reconstructed with iterative algorithms appear blotchy, plastic-looking, or unnatural, which poses problems for radiologists during image interpretation. To solve this problem, AI algorithms are now being used in CT image reconstruction.

In the AI domain, computers think and solve problems like humans. DL is a subset of machine learning, which is a subset of AI. It is not within the scope of this book (or this chapter) to describe the principles of AI. The interested reader should refer to an article by Seeram (2020) for further elaboration. One popular AI algorithm now used in CT image reconstruction is a DL algorithm called a *convolution neural network*: it is used in LD-CT to produce high-quality images comparable to those produced by iterative reconstruction algorithms. Two such DL-based algorithms approved by the US Food and Drug Administration in 2019 are the *Advanced Intelligent Clear-IQ Engine* (AiCE) from Canon Medical Systems and *TrueFidelity* from General Electric (GE) Healthcare. A further description of these two algorithms can be found in the paper by Seeram (2020).

Self-Assessment Questions will be based on each of the following Keywords and Concepts

- Projection profiles
- Sinogram
- Algorithm
- Image reconstruction
- Back-projection reconstruction
- Classical star blur
- Filtered back-projection reconstruction
- Convolution filter
- Iterative reconstruction (IR) algorithm
- Purpose of IR algorithms
- Artificial raw data
- Difference image
- Image quality criterion (IQC)
- IR loop
- Deep learning in CT image reconstruction

Challenge Questions

Answer the following questions to check your understanding of the materials studied.

True (T)/False (F)

1. Image reconstruction is the second step, following data acquisition, in the three-step process of creating CT images.
2. The output readings from the detectors are used to produce projection profiles.
3. The projection profiles from question 2 are used to reconstruct CT images.
4. Image reconstruction uses complex mathematics to create CT images using the attenuation values collected from the patient at various known locations of the x-ray tube and detectors.
5. The back-projection algorithm was one of the first algorithms used to reconstruct CT images.
6. The back-projection algorithm does not produce sharp images.
7. The back-projection algorithm produces blurred images called a *classical star pattern*.

8. The filtered back-projection algorithm produces sharp images and became the workhorse algorithm for decades.

9. The filtered back-projection algorithm does not use a convolution filter (digital filter) to sharpen images.

10. At low-dose CT, the filtered back-projection algorithm produces noisy images.

11. Iterative algorithms were developed to reduce noise on CT images and reduce the dose to patients when low doses are used.

12. Only three iterative algorithms are available from CT vendors.

13. Iterative algorithms use measured projection data to create the first estimate of the CT image.

14. The estimate from question 13 is forward projected (using mathematics) to create artificial raw data.

15. Artificial raw data is compared with measured data, and a difference is obtained to generate an updated image.

16. When using iterative algorithms, the user must determine an IQC.

17. When the difference is small enough to match the IQC, the iterative process stops, and the final CT image is created.

18. One example of an iterative algorithm is the *iterative loop*.

19. The final CT image created by the iterative process is much sharper than the initial CT image.

20. Adaptive iterative dose reduction (AIDR) is not an iterative algorithm.

Multiple Choice

1. In CT, projection profiles are:
   A. The shadow of the patient on the table
   B. Low energy x-ray photons from the patient
   C. Data sets used to develop the reconstruction algorithm
   D. X-ray transmission readings collected by the CT detectors

2. Projection profiles are used in CT to:
   A. Create CT images without a reconstruction algorithm
   B. Create images called sinograms
   C. Calculate the dose to the entrance surface of the patient
   D. Develop protocols for various body parts

3. Early CT image reconstruction algorithms:
   A. Required sinograms to produce diagnostic CT images
   B. Used projection profiles to create diagnostic CT images
   C. Did not use attenuation data from the patient to produce CT images
   D. Only required data collected over a rotation of 90°

4. Which of the following is a finite set of specific rules for solving a problem, such as the mathematical problem in CT?
   A. An algorithm
   B. A sinogram
   C. A computer flowchart
   D. A projection profile

5. The first algorithm used in CT was the:
   A. Iterative algorithm
   B. Filtered back-projection algorithm
   C. Analytic method called the Fourier transform
   D. Back-projection algorithm

6. A major problem with the first algorithm used in CT was:
   A. Image blur called the *classical star pattern*.
   B. Increased dose to the patient
   C. Incorrect coding by individuals lacking computer science skills
   D. That computers could not solve the problem when Hounsfield invented the first clinically useful CT scanner

7. Which of the following algorithms uses a convolution filter (digital filter) to solve the major problem of the first CT reconstruction algorithm?
   A. The back-projection algorithm
   B. The filtered back-projection algorithm
   C. The iterative algorithm
   D. The AIDR algorithm

8. Iterative algorithms were developed to:
   A. Reduce the noise from low-dose CT imaging
   B. Allow technologists to scan the patient very quickly
   C. Minimize the radiation dose to patients
   D. A and C are correct.

9. Which of the following is not an example of an iterative reconstruction algorithm?
   A. AIDR
   B. Filtered back-projection algorithm
   C. Model-based iterative reconstruction
   D. iDose

10. A major requirement of iterative algorithms is:
    A. High mAs with low kV settings
    B. Availability of an image quality criterion.
    C. Five iterative loops before a final CT image can be produced
    D. A smart CT operator

11. An important feature of iterative algorithms is:
    A. Artificial raw data
    B. Low-mAs technique
    C. Sinograms
    D. A mid-range computer system

12. The two data sets used in iterative reconstruction algorithms are essentially the:
    A. Initial image estimate and artificial raw data
    B. Patient scan parameters and protocol for the examination
    C. mAs and kV used for the scan
    D. Patient size and reconstruction field of view

13. Which of the following must be established by the user when using iterative reconstruction algorithms?
    A. mAs values
    B. Image spatial resolution
    C. Image quality criterion
    D. Approximate scan time for the particular examination

14. When using iterative reconstruction algorithms in CT, the iteration process stops:
    A. After the initial image estimate is forward projected
    B. After the artificial raw data is obtained
    C. When the difference between the artificial raw data and initial image estimate is computed
    D. When the difference between the artificial raw data and the initial image estimate is very small and meets the image quality criterion

15. Which is an AI-based algorithm now being used in CT image reconstruction?
    A. AIDR
    B. AiCE
    C. MBIR
    D. A and C are correct.

Short Answers

1. What is a projection profile in CT?
2. What is the result of using projection profiles without an image reconstruction algorithm?
3. Explain how the back-projection algorithm works. What is the major problem with this algorithm?
4. Describe how filtered back-projection works,

5. State the problem of using low-dose CT techniques and the filtered back-projection algorithm, and also state the solution to this problem.
6. What is meant by the term *iteration*? Describe the basic principles of an iterative algorithm used in CT.
7. State the main reason for using AI algorithms in CT image reconstruction. Which subset of machine learning (a subset of AI) now being used in CT image reconstruction? Give two CT vendor examples of these algorithms,

Answers to Challenge Questions

True/False

1. T	8. T	15. T
2. T	9. F	16. T
3. T	10. T	17. T
4. T	11. T	18. F
5. T	12. F	19. T
6. T	13. T	20. F
7. T	14. T	

Multiple Choice

1. D	6. A	11. A
2. B	7. B	12. A
3. A	8. D	13. C
4. A	9. B	14. D
5. D	10. B	15. B

Short Answer

1. A projection profile is generated from the attenuation values (from the patient) falling upon the CT detectors. The detectors convert x-ray photons into electrical signals called *projection profiles*.
2. If the projection profiles are used without an image reconstruction, a sinogram image is obtained. Sinogram images are not sectional CT images.
3. The back-projection algorithm was one of the first algorithms used in the early evolution of CT. The algorithm requires all projection

profiles collected to be back-projected. This back-projected data is then summed, and the result is a blurred image called a *classical star pattern*. The image is not diagnostic and cannot be used by radiologists to make a diagnosis.

4. The filtered back-projection algorithm removes the blurring inherent in the back-projection algorithm by first applying a digital filter to the projection profiles. This filter is called a *convolution filter*. These convolved filtered profiles are then back-projected. In the final process, the filtered profiles are summed to cancel negative and positive components and create a sectional CT image of the patient's anatomy being scanned. These reconstructed images are free of blurring and hence can be interpreted by radiologists to make a diagnosis. The filtered back-projection algorithm was used for decades until LD-CT received increasing attention because CT doses appeared to be increasing as the years progressed.

5. The problem with LD-CT with the new generation of CT scanners (multislice CT [MSCT] scanners) was that with the use of the filtered back-projection algorithm, the results were noisy images and streak artifacts. These limitations require other approaches to reduce the noise and not compromise image quality. Other approaches use smoothing digital filters and a new generation of CT reconstruction algorithms called *iterative reconstruction* (IR) algorithms.

6. The term *iteration* refers to "the repetition of a process or, more specifically, the repetition of a mathematical or computational procedure applied to the result of a previous application, typically as a means of obtaining successively closer approximations to the solution of a problem" (Google search, 2021).

7. The problems of long reconstruction times and images that appear blotchy when using iterative reconstruction algorithms with LD-CT techniques have been solved using DL algorithms. DL is a subset of machine learning, which is a subset of AI. Two such DL-based algorithms approved by the US Food and Drug Administration in 2019 are the Advanced Intelligent Clear-IQ Engine (AiCE) from Canon Medical Systems and TrueFidelity from General Electric (GE) Healthcare. These DL algorithms result in improved imaged quality compared with images reconstructed with iterative algorithms.

IDENTIFYING AREAS TO STUDY

A. Make a list of topics and/or questions that are still not clear to you after studying this chapter.

B. See the instructor for clarification and/or consolidation of the material.

7

CT Image Display, Storage, Communications, and Image Postprocessing

INTRODUCTION

Before attempting to answer these review questions, read the following brief notes.

CT image display and storage, picture archiving and communication systems (PACS), and CT image postprocessing belong to step 3 of the fundamental steps in CT imaging (Figure 7.1). While image display and storage include characteristics such as the display field of view (DFOV), spatial resolution, matrix size, bit depth, and windowing, PACS address the elements of electronic communications. Specifically, these include a definition of PACS, major system components, and two communication protocol standards: Digital Imaging and Communications in Medicine (DICOM), a communication standard for images; and Health-Level 7 (HL-7), a communication standard for text data. On the other hand, image postprocessing addresses digital

Computed Tomography: Physics and Technology A Self Assessment Guide,
Second Edition. Euclid Seeram.
© 2022 John Wiley & Sons Ltd. Published 2022 by John Wiley & Sons Ltd.

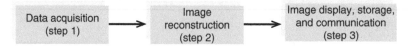

Figure 7.1   **Three essential steps in the production of a CT image.**

image processing operations. This chapter features only the post-processing operation of windowing: specifically, window width (WW) and window level (WL) operations used to manipulate image contrast and brightness, respectively. Typical WW and WL values for different tissues are 3000 and 500, 400 and 40, 80 and 40, and 1500 and −400 for temporal bone, soft tissues of the chest, brain, and lung, respectively.

Self-Assessment Questions will be based on each of the following Keywords and Concepts:

- Grayscale image
- Scan field of view (SFOV)
- Spatial resolution
- Matrix size
- Pixel size
- Bits per pixel
- Bit depth
- Image storage devices
- Electronic communication
- Meaning of the acronym PACS
- Meanings of the acronyms HIS and RIS
- System components of PACS
- Communication protocol standard
- Meanings of the acronyms DICOM and HL-7
- Image postprocessing definition
- Windowing and other synonymous terms
- WW and WL definitions
- Effect of WW and WL on image brightness and contrast, respectively
- Typical WW and WL values for different tissues
- Three-dimensional (3D) processing examples

Challenge Questions

Answer the following questions to check your understanding of the materials studied.

True (T)/False (F)

1. After the CT image has been reconstructed, the output from the CT computer is in digital (numerical) form.
2. Digital image data must be converted into grayscale images for viewing and interpretation by a trained human observer.
3. The scan field of view (SFOV) is the reconstruction circle located in the gantry where the patient is positioned for the scan.
4. The SFOV is the anatomical area being scanned.
5. The DFOV is the FOV seen on the viewing monitor.
6. The DFOV is greater than the SFOV.
7. Spatial resolution is characterized by the number of shades of gray seen in the displayed image.
8. The pixel size is related to the spatial resolution of an image.
9. The bit depth expresses the number of shades of gray each pixel of a CT image can assume.
10. The image postprocessing operation of windowing can be used to sharpen CT images.
11. The range of CT numbers is called the window width.
12. The center of the range of CT numbers is called the window level.

Multiple Choice

1. After CT image reconstruction, the reconstructed image (data) is:
   A. A grayscale image displayed on the viewing monitor
   B. A numerical image (digital image) displayed on the technologist viewing monitor to check the accuracy of the scan
   C. A digital image (numerical image) not displayed for interpretation
   D. Displayed on the medical physics monitor and used for quality control purposes
2. In digital image processing, a pixel is:
   A. A device that converts analog signals into digital data
   B. A contraction for the picture element
   C. An integer
   D. A shade of gray

3. In CT, a pixel is:
   A. A picture element on the display monitor
   B. A volume of tissue in the patient
   C. Another term for the attenuation coefficient
   D. An absorption value calculated after the radiation is transmitted through the patient
4. The circular region of the gantry aperture from which transmission data is collected during scanning is called:
   A. Display field of view (DFOV)
   B. Isocenter
   C. Scan FOV (SFOV)
   D. Circular aperture
5. The SFOV is also referred to as the:
   A. DFOV
   B. Reconstruction circle
   C. Voxel circle
   D. Matrix overlay
6. The exact center of the gantry aperture is referred to as the:
   A. SFOV
   B. DFOV
   C. Reconstruction center
   D. Isocenter
7. The DFOV is:
   A. The section of the scanned anatomy displayed on the viewing monitor
   B. The anatomical section positioned in the center of the gantry
   C. Also referred to as the display circle
   D. The matrix size
8. The DFOV is equal to the:
   A. Pixel size + matrix size
   B. Pixel size − matrix size
   C. Pixel size × matrix size
   D. Matrix size − pixel size
9. The spatial resolution of a CT image is related to the:
   A. Matrix size
   B. Reconstruction circle
   C. Isocenter
   D. Bit depth

10. Given that the DFOV is 25 cm and the matrix size is 512×512, the pixel size is:
    A. 0.5 cm
    B. 0.05 mm
    C. 0.5 mm
    D. 5.0 mm

11. The number of shades of gray that a single pixel can assume is determined by the:
    A. Bits per cm
    B. DFOV
    C. SFOV
    D. Bit depth

12. If n is the bit depth, the number of shades of gray that a pixel can assume is given by:
    A. 2^n
    B. 2×n
    C. 2n
    D. n^2

13. A CT image with a bit depth of 8 would have:
    A. 16 shades of gray
    B. 256 shades of gray
    C. 8 shades of gray
    D. 256/8 shades of gray

14. Which of the following general image processing operations is used to change the brightness and contrast of the displayed CT image?
    A. Windowing
    B. Edge enhancement
    C. Smoothing
    D. Contrast enhancement

15. CT images can only be stored on:
    A. Magnetic disks
    B. Optical disks
    C. Optical tape
    D. All are correct.

16. Which of the following uses formal rules to describe how to transmit or exchange image or textual data across a computer network?
    A. Radiology information system (RIS)
    B. Hospital information system (HIS)
    C. PACS
    D. DICOM and HL-7, respectively

17. Which of the following uses formal rules to describe how to transmit or exchange image data across a computer network?
    A. HL-7 communication protocol standard
    B. DICOM communication protocol standard
    C. HIS
    D. RIS

18. Which of the following uses formal rules to describe how to transmit or exchange textual data across a computer network?
    A. HL-7
    B. DICOM
    C. WORD processing
    D. RIS and HIS

19. The following is used to provide access to images remotely from a hospital/clinic PACS:
    A. Web server
    B. Web storage device
    C. Google search engine
    D. PACS controller

20. The range of CT numbers on a CT image is called the:
    A. Window width (WW)
    B. Window level (WL)
    C. Window center (WC)
    D. Attenuation values

21. The center or midpoint of the range of CT numbers on a CT image is called the:
    A. WW
    B. WL
    C. WC
    D. Linear attenuation coefficient (μ)

22. Which of the following change(s) the contrast of the image displayed on the viewing monitor?
    A. The WL control
    B. The kV setting on the control panel
    C. The mAs used for the examination
    D. The WW control

23. When the WW remains fixed and the WL is increased, the image changes from:
    A. Black to white
    B. White to black
    C. There is no change in the density of the image.
    D. Black to yellow

24. Which of the following is correct for the effect of the WW on image contrast?
    A. A wide WW results in a high-contrast image.
    B. A wide WW results in a low-contrast image.
    C. A narrow WW results in a low-contrast image.
    D. Contrast is optimized with a wide WW.

25. Setting a WW of 500 and a WL of 0 will result in the following:
    A. Those CT numbers above +250 appear white, while those below −250 appear black, and the gray scale extends between +250 and −250.
    B. Those CT numbers below −250 appear white, while those above +250 appear black, and the gray scale extends between +250 and +500.
    C. Those CT numbers above +500 appear black, while those below −500 appear white, and the gray scale extends between +250 and −250.
    D. Those CT numbers between +500 and −500 will be displayed as gray.

Short Answers

1. What are CT numbers, and why should they be displayed as shades of gray (grayscale)?
2. What is the difference between the SFOV and the DFOV?
3. Describe the fundamental characteristics that affect the spatial resolution of the CT image
4. What is the bit depth of the CT image? Explain how it affects the image gray scale.
5. How many gigabytes (GB) of storage are required to store a CT image having dimensions of 512×512×16 bits for 50 examinations performed in one day?
6. Define PACS, and describe the major components of PACS.
7. State two communication protocol standards in a PACS environment.

Answers to Challenge Questions

True/False

1. T	4. T	7. F
2. T	5. T	8. T
3. T	6. F	9. T
10. F		

Multiple Choice

1. C	10. C	19. A
2. B	11. D	20. A
3. A	12. A	21. B
4. C	13. B	22. D
5. B	14. A	23. B
6. D	15. D	24. B
7. A	16. D	25. A
8. C	17. B	
9. A	18. A	

Short Answer

1. CT numbers are computed from the attenuation data collected from the patient. The image is therefore available on the computer as digital numbers. These numbers must be converted into grayscale images for display on a viewing monitor to be interpreted by a human observer, usually a radiologist. Radiologists are usually well versed in viewing grayscale images for diagnostic interpretation (instead of color images or numerical images).

2. The patient is first positioned in the gantry in preparation for scanning. The technologist selects the best positioning of the body part and ensures that this part is exposed appropriately to the radiation beam. The SFOV is also referred to as the *reconstruction circle*. It exactly defines the anatomical body part to be accurately scanned. After scanning, the image is displayed on a viewing monitor for interpretation. This is the DFOV. The DFOV can be equal to or less than the SFOV.

3. Spatial resolution refers to the sharpness of the image. For digital images, the spatial resolution depends on the size of the pixel, which can be calculated by knowing the FOV and the matrix size. In general, the smaller the pixel size, the better the spatial resolution. The pixel size can be calculated using the following algebraic expression:

Pixel Size = FOV/Matrix Size

This means that for the same FOV, the larger the matrix size, the smaller the pixel size, and the better the spatial resolution of the CT image.

4. Each pixel in a CT image can assume a range of gray shades. The image can have 256 (2^8), 512 (2^9), 1024 (2^{10}), 2048 (2^{11}), or 4096 (2^{12}) different grayscale values. As noted, these numbers are represented as bits, and therefore a CT image can be characterized by the number of bits per pixel; that is, a CT image can have 8, 9, 10, 11, or 12 bits per pixel. In this case, a CT image consists of a series of bit planes, referred to as the *bit depth*. The numerical value of the pixel represents the brightness level of the image at that pixel position.

5. A CT image of 512×512×2 bytes will require 0.5 megabytes (MB). To store images from a CT examination consisting of 50 images would require 25 MB (0.5×50) of storage capacity. A workload of 50 examinations in a single day would require 1.25 GB of storage capacity.

6. PACS is an electronic communication system coupled to the image acquisition system (in this case, the CT scanner) that is characterized by a number of electronic communication technologies, not only to store and archive CT images but also to transmit images to remote locations using computer networks. Interfaces are used to couple devices in the entire system. Images from the CT scanner are sent to the PACS controller, which includes a database and servers such as the image and archive servers as well as an archival storage device. The PACS is integrated with the RIS and HIS. Communication of images and text data are accommodated using communication protocol standards, such as DICOM and HL-7. While DICOM addresses communication of images, HL-7 primarily deals with the communication of text data.

IDENTIFYING AREAS TO STUDY

A. Make a list of topics and/or questions that are still not clear to you after studying this chapter.

B. See the instructor for clarification and/or consolidation of the material.

8

Multislice CT: Fundamental Principles

PRIOR READING ASSIGNMENT

Before attempting to answer these review questions, read the following summary of essential principles of multislice CT (MSCT).

MSCT is a *state-of-the-art* type of CT used today, and therefore the following brief notes are essential to ensure wise use of these scanners and prepare for examinations. These scanners are based on the principles and concepts described in the past seven chapters; however, there are special technical principles that must be considered. This chapter will address the *principles and technology of MSCT*.

The *evolution of CT* is marked by continuous developments of the technical innovations intended to improve data acquisition; image reconstruction; and image display, storage, and communications for the purpose of improving patient care and management. The evolution of the *first CT scanner* invented by *Godfrey Hounsfield* (which only scanned the head) led to the introduction of other scanners for

Computed Tomography: Physics and Technology A Self Assessment Guide,
Second Edition. Euclid Seeram.
© 2022 John Wiley & Sons Ltd. Published 2022 by John Wiley & Sons Ltd.

scanning the entire body. These scanners have been popularly referred to as *conventional CT* (CCT), *single-slice CT* (SSCT), and MSCT. While CCT involves scanning a single slice in a single breath-hold in a *stop-and-go* or *slice-by-slice fashion*, SSCT acquires volume data sets much faster than CCT by using a *one-dimensional (1D) detector array* that rotates continuously while the patient moves through the gantry to cover the entire length of tissue. The path traced by the x-ray beam coupled with *patient translation* describes a beam geometry referred to as *spiral/helical* CT. Finally, MSCT was developed to acquire volume data sets much faster than SSCT scanners using a two-dimensional (2D) detector array and spiral/helical beam geometry. There are two types of 2D detectors: *matrix array detectors* and *adaptive array detectors*.

There are several technical requirements for *volume scanning*, including continuous rotation of the x-ray tube and detectors, continuous motion of the table through the gantry aperture during scanning, increased electrical loadability of the x-ray tube, higher cooling rates of the x-ray tube, special algorithms related to spiral/helical scanning, and increased memory storage for the huge amounts of data collected during MSCT scanning. Continuous rotation of the x-ray tube and detectors during scanning is made possible by using *slip rings* (electromechanical devices consisting of circular electrical conductive rings and brushes that transmit electrical energy across a rotating interface). While some CT vendors use a *low-voltage slip ring*, others use a *high-voltage slip ring*.

The slice geometry is somewhat different for SSCT and MSCT. While in SSCT, a *planar section* (section perpendicular to the long axis of the body) is obtained per revolution of the x-ray tube and detectors; this is not the case with MSCT, since the patient is moving through the gantry as the tube and detectors rotate continuously around the patient. In MSCT, a planar section is not obtained, and therefore it must be computed. A planar section is required by the reconstruction algorithm and is computed using the acquisition data by *interpolation,* a mathematical technique for estimating the value of a function from known values from either side of it. Without interpolation, streaking artifacts in the image are seen. Interpolation removes these artifacts and occurs before image reconstruction. Two types of interpolation are used: 360° Z-interpolation (Z-axis = longitudinal axis of the patient) and 180° Z-interpolation. The latter produces a much sharper image than the former.

Two types of detectors are used in MSCT: the matrix array detector and the adaptive array detector (Figure 8.1). The *detector configuration* is an important consideration when using these systems. The detector configuration refers to how the detector elements can be combined (*binned*) to produce the slice thickness needed for the examination. While *wide collimation* results in thicker slices, *narrow collimation* produces thin slices resulting in improved image sharpness. In order to reduce the noise in thin slice imaging, the dose must be increased.

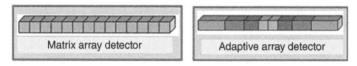

Matrix array detector | Adaptive array detector

Figure 8.1 **Two types of MSCT detector arrays.**

In MSCT systems, the pitch is defined by the International Electrotechnical Commission (IEC) as:

Pitch (P) = the distance (d) the table travels per rotation/ the total collimation (W)

That is,

P = d/W

The total collimation, on the other hand, is equal to the number of slices (M) multiplied by the collimated slice thickness (S). Algebraically, the pitch is now expressed as

P = d/W or P = d/M × S

It is important to note that the higher the pitch, the faster the imaging time and the lower the dose to the patient. However, image quality is compromised compared to the use of lower pitch, which also involves a higher dose to the patient.

Selectable scan parameters can be used in MSCT systems to optimize the dose to the patient. These parameters fall into two categories: primary and secondary selectable scan parameters. The former include the mA, kV, automatic exposure control (AEC), pitch, scan time, and scan length; the latter include the slice thickness, field of view (FOV), reconstruction algorithm, reconstruction interval, spatial and contrast resolution, and geometric efficiency.

Self-Assessment Questions will be based on each of the following Keywords and Concepts

- Evolution of CT
- Stop-and-go or slice-by-slice data acquisition
- Spiral or helical data acquisition
- Volume data acquisition
- One-dimensional (1D) detector array
- Two-dimensional detector (2D) array
- Matrix array detectors
- Adaptive array detectors
- Technical requirements for volume scanning
- Slip ring technology
- Slice geometry for SSCT
- Planar section
- Slice geometry for MSCT
- Interpolation
- 360° Z-interpolation
- 180° Z-interpolation
- Detector configuration
- Narrow collimation
- Wide collimation
- Pitch for MSCT
- Selectable scan parameters

Challenge Questions

Answer the following questions to check your understanding of the materials studied.

True (T)/False (F)

1. Godfrey Hounsfield invented the first clinically useful CT scanner for examining the head only.

2. Early CT scanners, referred to as CCT scanners, are based on scanning only one slice per single breath-hold.

3. SSCT scanners overcome the limitations imposed by CCT scanners and can therefore scan the patient much faster than CCT scanners.

4. SSCT scanners use 2D detector arrays to collect more than one slice per revolution of the x-ray tube and detectors.

5. SSCT scanners provide notable improvements in 3D images compared to CCT scanners.

6. MSCT scanners use 2D detector arrays to collect more than one slice per revolution of the x-ray tube and detectors.

7. MSCT scanners acquire volume data sets and have a much faster volume coverage speed than SSCT scanners.

8. Since MSCT scanners use 2D detector arrays, they are also called multi-detector CT (MDCT) scanners.

9. The terms *spiral* and *helical* refer to the path traced by the x-ray beam as the patient moves through the gantry.

10. While Canon Medical Systems use the term *spiral*, Siemens Healthineers uses the term *helical* to describe MSCT scanners.

11. Matrix array detectors are based on the use of equal-sized detector elements in the detector array.

12. Adaptive array detectors consist of equal pairs of detector elements.

13. MSCT scanners use slip ring technology to enable the table to move simultaneously as the x-ray tube and detectors rotate continuously around the patient.

14. MSCT scanners use slip ring technology to enable continuous rotation of the x-ray tube and detectors around the patient.

15. Interpolation is an essential requirement in MSCT before image reconstruction.

16. Without interpolation, images have streak artifacts.

17. When using MSCT scanners, the term *detector configuration* refers to the ways detector elements are binned (combined) to produce the desired slice thickness.

18. A narrow collimation in MSCT scanning will result in sharper images (compared to wider collimation) but increased noise.

19. 180° Z-interpolation approaches in MSCT scanners generate thinner slices from planar sections than 360° Z-interpolation approaches.

20. The algebraic expression for the pitch (P) in MSCT scanning is a ratio of the distance (d) the table travels per rotation to the total collimation (W) represented as P = d/W.

Multiple Choice

1. The first clinically useful CT scanner was restricted to scanning only the:
   A. Head
   B. Chest and abdomen
   C. Extremities
   D. All are correct.
2. The method of scanning a patient in CCT scanners involves:
   A. Scanning two slices per revolution of the x-ray tube and detectors
   B. Moving the table through the gantry aperture during one revolution
   C. Scanning one slice per revolution, stopping, advancing the patient for the next slice, scanning the patient, and then stopping and going (repeating) again
   D. Scanning two slices of tissue per revolution of the x-ray tube and detectors
3. Which of the following methods of data acquisition is characteristic of SSCT scanners?
   A. Stop-and-go data acquisition
   B. Slice-by-slice data acquisition
   C. Moving the table to scan a volume of tissue
   D. Moving the table while the x-ray tube and detectors rotate simultaneously around the patient, using a 1D detector array to collect one slice per revolution
4. Which of the following data acquisition methods is characteristic of state-of-the-art MSCT scanners?
   A. Stop-and-go data acquisition
   B. Slice-by-slice data acquisition
   C. Moving the table to scan a volume of tissue using a 1D detector array that rotates at the same time the table moves through the gantry aperture
   D. Move the table while the x-ray tube and detectors rotate simultaneously around the patient, using a 2D detector array to collect multiple slices per revolution

5. Which of the following describes the *spiral/helical* scanning using 2D detectors arrays characteristic of MSCT scanners?
   A. The path traced by the x-ray tube and detectors as the patient moves through the gantry aperture during data acquisition
   B. The use of 2D detector arrays during data acquisition
   C. The translation of the table with the patient in the supine position while the x-ray tube and detectors remain stationary
   D. All are correct.

6. The overall goal of spiral/helical CT scanning is to:
   A. Increase the patient speed through the scanner aperture
   B. Increase the speed of the rotation of the x-ray tube
   C. Increase the volume coverage speed performance
   D. Decrease the scan time

7. The cable wrap-around problem in CCT is eliminated by which of the following?
   A. High-capacity x-ray tube
   B. High-frequency generator
   C. Slip ring technology
   D. Spiral/helical weighting algorithm

8. In spiral/helical CT scanning, an *interpolation algorithm* is needed to:
   A. Produce a planar section (data set)
   B. Reconstruct the final CT image in the volume
   C. Remove streaking artifacts caused by the presence of metal
   D. Remove beam-hardening artifacts

9. The purpose of the slip ring in a spiral/helical CT scanner is to:
   A. Remove ring artifacts
   B. Allow the table to move only 10 cm
   C. Provide continuous rotation of the x-ray tube and detectors so that a volume of tissue can be scanned
   D. Provide increased voltage to the x-ray tube

10. One of the most noticeable differences between single-slice and multislice CT systems is the:
    A. Detector design
    B. Computer system
    C. Image display subsystem
    D. Thickness of the section

11. For multislice CT scanning, the slice thickness is determined by:
    A. The number of channels in the detector design
    B. The data acquisition system (DAS)

    C. The number of detector elements grouped together (binned)

    D. All are correct.

12. Which term describes the ratio of the table travels per revolution of the x-ray tube and detectors to the collimation beam width?

    A. Dose-length product

    B. Pitch ratio

    C. Scan ratio

    D. Tilt ratio

13. The definition of pitch ratio in a multislice scanner, as defined by the International Electrotechnical Commission, states that:

    A. $P =$ distance the table travels per rotation (d)/total collimation (W)

    B. $P = d + W$

    C. $P = d \times W$

    D. $P = W/d$

14. For spiral/helical CT scanning, which of the following pitch ratios produces the best image quality?

    A. $1:1$

    B. $2:1$

    C. $3:1$

    D. $6:1$

15. Which of the following pitch ratios will result in the largest volume coverage in the fastest time?

    A. $1:1$

    B. $2:1$

    C. $4:1$

    D. $6:1$

16. Which of the following pitch ratios will result in the highest dose to the patient?

    A. $1:1$

    B. $2:1$

    C. $4:1$

    D. $6:1$

17. In spiral/helical CT scanning, the *effective mAs* can be defined as:

    A. Effective mAs = kilovolts/pitch

    B. Effective mAs = mAs + pitch

    C. Effective mAs = mAs/pitch

    D. Effective mAs = pitch/kilovolts

18. In MSCT scanning, the following is considered a primary scan parameter (PSP):
    A. Reconstruction algorithm
    B. Automatic exposure control
    C. Spatial resolution
    D. Geometric efficiency

19. In MSCT scanning, the following is considered a secondary scan parameter (SSP):
    A. Reconstruction algorithm
    B. Pitch
    C. mA
    D. kV

20. In CT scanning, which term describes dose reduction without compromising image quality according to the ALARA (as low as reasonably achievable) philosophy?
    A. Computed tomography dose index
    B. Optimization
    C. Pitch ratio
    D. Selectable reconstruction parameter

Short Answers

1. Explain what is meant by *spiral/helical* beam geometry in MSCT scanning.
2. What is the major difference between SSCT and MSCT scanning?
3. What is the difference between matrix detectors and adaptive detectors used in MSCT scanners?
4. What is volume CT? List the primary technical requirements for MSCT volume scanning.
5. Outline the main difference between low-voltage and high-voltage slip ring technology used in MSCT scanners.
6. Explain the difference between the slice geometry for SSCT and MSCT scanning
7. What is the meaning of interpolation, and why is it an important first step in MSCT scanning?
8. Compare 360° Z-interpolation and 180° Z-interpolation in MSCT scanners.
9. State the meaning of the term *detector configuration* for MSCT scanners.

10. Write out the algebraic expression for the pitch in MSCT scanners as provided by the International Electrotechnical Commission (IEC).
11. What are selectable scan parameters?

Answers to Challenge Questions

True/False

1. T	8. T	15. T
2. T	9. T	16. T
3. T	10. F	17. T
4. F	11. T	18. T
5. T	12. F	19. T
6. T	13. F	20. T
7. T	14. T	

Multiple Choice

1. A	8. A	15. D
2. C	9. C	16. A
3. D	10. A	17. C
4. D	11. C	18. B
5. A	12. B	19. A
6. C	13. A	20. B
7. C	14. A	

Short Answers

1. The term *beam geometry* as used in CT refers to the size, shape, and motion of the x-ray beam emanating from the x-ray tube and passing through the patient to strike the detector array, which collects radiation attenuation data from the patient. In MSCT, the beam geometry is described as spiral or helical (spiral/helical), which means that the path traced by the x-ray beam as the patient moves through the CT gantry aperture describes a spiral or a helix. The advantage of this beam geometry is that it increases the volume coverage speed during the scanning of the patient.
2. The major difference between SSCT and MSCT is based on the type of detector array used. While SSCT scanners use a 1D detector array to collect one slice per revolution of the tube and detectors, MSCT scanners use a 2D detector array to collect multiple slices (64, 128, 256, or 320, for example) per revolution of the tube and detectors during scanning.

3. A significant physical difference between matrix array and adaptive array detectors used in CT (see Figure 8.1) is the design. While a matrix array detector consists of equal detector elements, adaptive array detectors are designed with pairs of elements that are equal: for example, the central two elements are equal or the two closest to the central ones are equal.

4. The term *volume CT* denotes that a volume of tissue is acquired during a single breath-hold (as opposed to a single slice, as is the case with SSCT). Volume CT data acquisition must meet the following two essential technical requirements:

   A. The use of slip ring technology to allow the continuous rotation of the x-ray tube and detectors

   B. The continuous motion of the table during data acquisition

5. The major difference between a low-voltage slip ring and a high-voltage slip-ring CT scanner is illustrated in Figure 8.2. While in the former, the low-voltage AC (alternating current) is sent to the slip ring; in the latter, the low-voltage AC must first be increased (a function of the high-voltage generator) and subsequently sent to the slip ring. Additionally, with the high-voltage approach, the x-ray generator does not rotate with the x-ray tube and detectors. Some CT vendors use the former approach, while others use the latter.

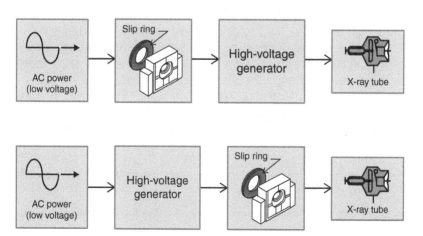

Figure 8.2 The major difference between low-voltage and high-voltage sling CT scanners (see the answer to question 5).

6. The slice geometry for SSCT and MSCT data acquisition is shown in Figure 8.3. While a planar section is acquired in SSCT (Figure 8.3a), a non-planar section is acquired in the MSCT approach (Figure 8.3b). The reconstruction algorithm used in CT scanners requires a planar section that generates consistent data.

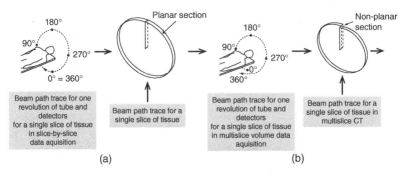

Figure 8.3   The major difference between the slice geometry for SSCT and MSCT data acquisition (see the answer to question 6).

7. Interpolation is a mathematical procedure for estimating the value of a function from known values on either side of it (as illustrated in Figure 8.4). Interpolation must be done first (before image reconstruction) to generate a planar section, thus satisfying the algorithm requirements. Without interpolation, streak artifacts will be seen in images. Interpolation eliminates these streak artifacts.

8. Two types of interpolation are used in MSCT: 360° linear interpolation (360° Z-interpolation) and a180° linear interpolation (180° Z-interpolation). The advantage of the latter approach is that thinner and sharper images can be produced compared to the former approach.

9. The term *detector configuration* as applied to MSCT refers to different ways that detector elements can be combined (binned) electronically to produce the desired slice thickness required for the examination.

10. In MSCT, the pitch (P) is defined by the International Electrotechnical Commission as the distance the table travels per rotation (d) divided by the total collimation (W). The algebraic expression is P = d/W

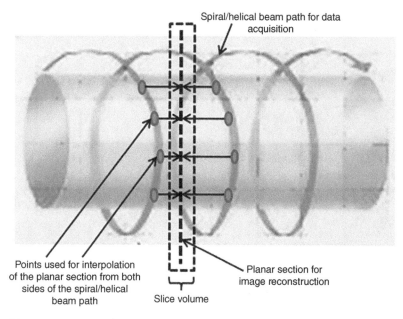

Spiral/helical beam path for data
acquisition

Points used for interpolation
of the planar section from both
sides of the spiral/helical
beam path

Planar section for
image reconstruction

Slice volume

Figure 8.4   Interpolation creates a planar section before image
reconstruction. This is a fundamental requirement for
MSCT scanners.

11. Selectable scan parameters fall into two groups: PSPs and SSPs.
PSPs include mA, kV, AEC, automatic voltage selection, pitch,
scan time, and scan length. SSPs, on the other hand, include
slice thickness, FOV, reconstruction algorithm, reconstruction
interval, spatial resolution, contrast resolution, and geometric
efficiency.

IDENTIFYING AREAS TO STUDY

A. Make a list of topics and/or questions that are still not clear to you
after studying this chapter.

B. See the instructor for clarification and/or consolidation of the
material.

9

Image Quality in CT

PRIOR READING ASSIGNMENT	85	IDENTIFYING AREAS TO STUDY	95
Challenge Questions	88		

PRIOR READING ASSIGNMENT

Before attempting to answer these review questions, read the following brief summary notes about the essentials of image quality in CT.

Image quality in CT can be described in terms of five physical parameters: spatial resolution, contrast resolution, temporal resolution, noise, and artifacts.

Spatial resolution is the ability of the CT scanner to resolve closely spaced objects that are significantly different from their background or to show small objects that have high subject contrast. Image spatial resolution means sharp, high detail images. Since CT is a digital imaging modality, images are digital, and the degree of detail depends on the matrix size, field of view (FOV), and slice thickness. The *matrix* is made up of horizontal and vertical pixels (picture elements), and the

Computed Tomography: Physics and Technology A Self Assessment Guide,
Second Edition. Euclid Seeram.
© 2022 John Wiley & Sons Ltd. Published 2022 by John Wiley & Sons Ltd.

pixel size determines the sharpness of the image. Smaller pixels (for the same FOV) will produce sharper images. The *pixel size* is equal to the FOV divided by the matrix size. Additionally, there are two features of spatial resolution in CT: the *in-plane spatial resolution* (the resolution in the X-Y axis of the patient) and the *cross-plane spatial resolution* (the resolution along the Z-axis of the patient). Spatial resolution is expressed as *line pairs per centimeter* (lp/cm) or *line pairs per millimeter* (lp/mm). Factors affecting the in-plane spatial resolution are the slice thickness, size of the detector cell, collimation, reconstruction algorithm, reconstruction filters, pixel size, FOV, and other factors such as the focal spot size, scanner geometry, and so on. The cross-plane resolution is often described by the term *slice sensitivity profile* (SSP), which is a plot of the beam intensity as a function of the location along the Z-axis (SSP curve). The slice thickness can be obtained by measuring the *full width at half the maximum* of the SSP curve. The resolution in the Z-axis is much better in spiral/helical CT scanning than conventional CT scanners.

Contrast resolution (sometimes referred to as *contrast sensitivity*) is the ability of the CT scanner to resolve small differences in soft tissues: that is, to show low-contrast tissues whose density is slightly different than the background. The visibility of structures in the image is highly affected by noise (described in the next paragraph). Factors (under the operator's control) affecting the contrast resolution include kV, mA, scan speed, FOV, reconstruction algorithm, and slice thickness. mA and kV control the amount of photons incident on the detector. More photons mean less image noise but increased dose to the patient. Increasing the slice thickness will improve contrast resolution. Increasing the FOV with a smaller matrix size (larger pixels) will improve contrast resolution. Compared to the filtered back-projection (FBP) algorithm, iterative reconstruction (IR) algorithms improve contrast resolution. A graph that shows the measured contrast plotted as a function of the detectable diameter of an object is referred to as a *contrast-detail diagram*. This diagram also characterizes the resolution of the CT scanner.

Temporal resolution is the ability of the scanner to freeze the motion of the scanned object. It is important in cardiac imaging. A major factor affecting temporal resolution is the scan speed. By increasing the scan speed, it is possible to freeze the motion of objects such as the beating heart, for example.

Noise in CT refers to random variations in the CT image. A large variation of CT numbers of a water phantom means that the image is very noisy. Several factors affect noise: mA, kV, filtration, slice thickness, pixel size, detector efficiency, and IR algorithms. More photons reaching the detector will produce less noise but more dose to the patient. Therefore, operators must work within the ALARA (as low as reasonably achievable) and use the lowest dose possible and not compromise image quality.

Artifacts in CT (Figure 9.1) have been defined by Dr. Jiang Hsieh, PhD, the chief medical physicist at GE Healthcare, as "any discrepancy between the reconstructed CT numbers in the image and the true attenuation coefficients of the object." Artifacts appear on CT images as streaks, bands of shading, rings, and other features such as moiré patterns and basket weave. CT artifacts are caused by patient motion, metal, beam hardening, and partial volume effects.

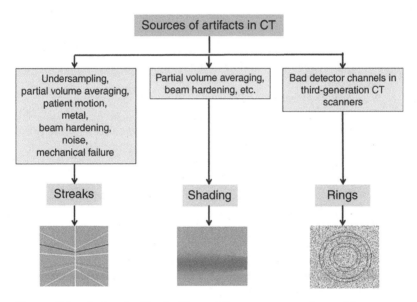

Figure 9.1   A simple illustration of the sources and graphic appearance of typical artifacts in CT.

Self-Assessment Questions will be based on each of the following Keywords and Concepts

- Physical parameters characterizing image quality
- Spatial resolution definition

- Factors affecting spatial resolution
- Contrast resolution definition
- Factors affecting contrast resolution
- Noise definition
- Factors affecting noise
- Artifact definition
- Sources of artifacts
- Appearance of artifacts

Challenge Questions

Answer the following questions to check your understanding of the materials studied.

True (T)/False (F)

1. Image quality in CT includes spatial resolution and contrast resolution only.
2. A technical parameter of image quality in CT is noise.
3. Artifacts are related to CT image quality.
4. A streaking artifact on a CT image is typically caused by the presence of metal in the patient.
5. Beam-hardening artifacts appear as a shading artifact on a CT image.
6. A bad detector element can create artifacts that appear as rings on CT images.
7. Partial volume averaging and patient motion will create ring artifacts on CT images.
8. Contrast resolution is affected by noise.
9. Spatial resolution is not influenced by factors affecting noise.
10. Temporal resolution refers to the scanner's ability to freeze motion.
11. Temporal resolution is not a significant parameter in cardiac CT.
12. Increasing the mA for an examination will decrease the noise but increase the dose to the patient.
13. More photons falling on the detector will increase the image noise and reduce the dose to the patient.
14. A ring artifact is due to a detector channel not working (out of order) for CT scanners that use third-generation beam geometry.

Multiple Choice

1. Which of the following image quality parameters relate to the number of photons falling on the detector to create an image?
   A. Noise
   B. Spatial resolution
   C. Contrast resolution
   D. All are correct.

2. An image quality parameter that refers to the CT scanner freezing the motion of the heart is:
   A. Noise
   B. Contrast resolution
   C. Artifact suppression
   D. Temporal resolution

3. The ability of the CT scanner to show low-contrast tissues whose density is slightly different than the background is called:
   A. Spatial resolution
   B. Contrast resolution
   C. Noise
   D. Temporal resolution

4. Any discrepancy between the reconstructed CT numbers in the image and the true attenuation coefficients of the object is referred to as:
   A. Image noise
   B. Spatial un-sharpness
   C. Contrast degradation
   D. Artifacts

5. Which of the following technical parameters does not affect spatial resolution in CT?
   A. Matrix size
   B. FOV
   C. kV
   D. Pixel size

6. The cross-plane resolution in CT is the resolution in the:
   A. X-axis of the patient
   B. Z-axis of the patient
   C. Y-axis of the patient
   D. X–Y axis of the patient

7. The in-plane spatial resolution in CT is the:
   A. Resolution in the X–Y axis of the patient
   B. Resolution in the Z-axis of the patient

    C. Resolution in the Y-axis of the patient

    D. Resolution on the X-axis of the patient

8. Which of the following algebraic expressions is correct?

    A. Pixel size (P) = Matrix size (M)/Field-of-view (FOV)

    B. P = M×FOV

    C. P = M+FOV

    D. P = FOV/M

9. For the same FOV, which matrix size will produce the sharpest image?

    A. 128×128

    B. 256×256

    C. 512×512

    D. 1024×1024

10. Which of the following is obtained by measuring the full width at half the maximum of the SSP?

    A. Slice thickness

    B. Pixel size

    C. Contrast resolution

    D. FOV

11. Line pairs per centimeter (lp/cm) or line pairs per millimeter (lp/mm) is used to express:

    A. Spatial resolution

    B. Contrast resolution

    C. Noise

    D. Temporal resolution

12. Contrast resolution in CT refers to the:

    A. Ability of the scanner to image different-size objects in the patient

    B. Ability of the scanner to image small differences in tissue contrast

    C. An image with different shades of gray

    D. Ability of the scanner to show small objects against a uniform background

13. Another term for contrast resolution is:

    A. Contrast curve

    B. Contrast sensitivity

    C. CT numbers

    D. Attenuation values

14. A graph illustrating the measured contrast plotted as a function of the detectable diameter of an object in the patient or phantom is referred to as a:
    A. Contrast-noise diagram
    B. High-contrast diagram
    C. Contrast-detail diagram
    D. Low-contrast sensitivity curve
15. The method used to characterize the resolution capabilities of a CT scanner is:
    A. A contrast-detail diagram
    B. Ask the CT vendor.
    C. Ask the CT technologist.
    D. Read the quality control notes of the medical physicist.
16. The following factors affect the contrast resolution in CT *except*:
    A. FOV
    B. Size of the detector cell
    C. mA and kV
    D. Slice thickness
17. Temporal resolution is the ability of the CT scanner to:
    A. Show the timing of object motion on the patient
    B. Show small differences in tissue contrast
    C. Freeze the motion of the scanned body part, such as the beating heart in cardiac CT imaging
    D. Demonstrate how fast the heart beats when the patient is in the scanner
18. A large variation of CT numbers from point to point in an image of a water phantom is defined as :
    A. Linearity
    B. Contrast resolution
    C. Uniformity
    D. Noise
19. Noise in CT is affected by all of the following *except*:
    A. Size of the x-ray tube focal spot
    B. Slice thickness
    C. mA and kV
    D. FOV
20. Lower noise is obtained when detail is increased by:
    A. Increasing the slice thickness
    B. Increasing the mA

C. Using iterative reconstruction instead of the filtered back projection reconstruction algorithm
D. All are correct.

21. Which of the following slice thicknesses will result in more noise in the image, all other factors being held constant?
A. 3 mm
B. 4 mm
C. 6 mm
D. 8 mm

22. Which of the following results in beam hardening?
A. Filtering the x-ray beam
B. Increasing the kV and mA
C. Iterative reconstruction algorithm
D. Smaller matrix sizes

23. A streaking artifact in CT is produced by:
A. Partial volume averaging
B. Metal in the patient
C. Patient motion
D. All are correct.

24. A ring artifact from a CT scanner using a third-generation beam geometry is caused by:
A. A bad detector channel
B. Beam hardening
C. Partial volume averaging
D. Metal in the patient

25. A shading artifact in CT is usually produced by:
A. Partial volume averaging
B. Beam hardening
C. Noise
D. A and B are correct.

Short Answers

1. What are the five physical characteristics of CT image quality? Define each of them.
2. What are the approximate spatial and contrast resolution values for a CT scanner?
3. Identify and explain the factors affecting spatial resolution in CT.
4. Identify and explain the factors affecting contrast resolution in CT.
5. Identify and explain several factors affecting noise in CT.

6. What is an artifact?
7. Identify several sources of artifacts, and describe their typical appearance on CT images.

Answers to Challenge Questions

True/False

1. F	4. T	7. F
2. T	5. T	8. T
3. T	6. T	9. T
10. T		
11. F	13. F	
12. T	14. T	

Multiple Choice

1. A	10. A	19. A
2. D	11. A	20. D
3. B	12. B	21. D
4. D	13. B	22. A
5. C	14. C	23. D
6. B	15. A	24. A
7. A	16. B	25. D
8. A	17. C	
9. D	18. D	

Short Answers

1. The five physical characteristics of CT image quality are spatial resolution, contrast resolution, noise, temporal resolution, and artifacts. Spatial resolution is the ability of the CT scanner to resolve close-spaced objects that are significantly different from their background. It is also the ability of the scanner to show small objects that have high subject contrast. These definitions indicate that the scanner can show image detail or image sharpness. Contrast resolution refers to the ability of the scanner to show small differences in tissue contrast. Noise is the random variation of CT numbers in the image. Temporal resolution is the ability of the scanner to freeze organ motion, such as the beating heart. Finally, an artifact is defined as distortions or errors in the image that are not related to the object being imaged.

2. The spatial resolution of a CT scanner depends on the imaging mode. While it is 10–14 lp/cm in standard imaging mode, 20 lp/cm is possible in high-resolution imaging mode. The contrast resolution in CT is 4 mm at 0.5%. Furthermore, CT can detect density differences ranging from 0.25 to 0.5%. CT has better contrast resolution than radiography, which can differentiate 10 mm objects compared to 4 mm objects for CT.

3. Factors affecting spatial resolution in CT include slice thickness, detector cell size, collimation, reconstruction algorithm, pixel size and FOV, reconstruction filters, and other factors such as focal spot size and scanner beam geometry. Thin slices, smaller detectors, and smaller focal spots result in sharper images. Additionally, narrow pre-detector collimation improves image sharpness. A bone algorithm produces sharper images than the standard reconstruction algorithm. Iterative reconstruction algorithms produce sharper images than the older reconstruction algorithm called the FBP algorithm. For the same FOV, smaller pixel sizes produce sharper images.

4. Several factors affect contrast resolution in CT. These include the kV, mA, scan speed (secs), reconstruction algorithm, and slice thickness. Lower mA and kV result in fewer photons striking the detector, and hence more noise is inherent in the images, resulting in grainy images that affect contrast resolution. Increased slice thickness and larger FOV result in improved contrast resolution. Compared to the FBP reconstruction algorithm, iterative reconstruction algorithms improve contrast resolution in low-dose CT scanning.

5. Noise is affected by several technical factors that determine the number of photons used to create the image. Among these are the mA, kV, beam filtration, slice thickness, detector efficiency, pixel size, and iterative reconstruction algorithms. While higher kV and mA values produce more photons and reduce noise in the image, greater beam filtration reduces the number of photons falling on the detector and therefore creates more image noise. Increased slice thickness, increased pixel size, and greater detector efficiency result in less image noise. With low-dose CT, iterative reconstruction algorithms improve image noise compared to the FBP algorithm.

6. An artifact is defined by Dr. Jiang Hsieh, PhD (senior medical physicist for GE Healthcare) as "any discrepancy between the

reconstructed CT numbers in the image and the true attenuation coefficients of the object." As noted by Dr. Hsieh, this definition "implies anything that causes an incorrect measurement of transmission readings by the detectors on an inconsistency between the measurement and reconstruction will result in an image artifact."

7. The sources of CT artifacts and the typical effects on images are summarized in Figure 9.1.

IDENTIFYING AREAS TO STUDY

A. Make a list of topics and/or questions that are still not clear to you after studying this chapter.

B. See the instructor for clarification and/or consolidation of the material.

10

Dose Optimization in CT

PRIOR READING ASSIGNMENT

Before attempting to answer these review questions, read the following brief summary notes of the essentials of dose optimization in CT.

Dose optimization in CT incorporates several topics such as radiation risks, radiation protection philosophy, dose metrics, factors affecting the dose, and optimization of radiation protection. Each of these will be reviewed briefly.

The motivation for optimizing the dose in CT stems from the known risks of radiation exposure to humans. These risks have been categorized into stochastic risks and deterministic risks. *Stochastic effects* are random: that is, the probability of their occurrence depends on the dose received and increases as the dose increases. There is no threshold dose for stochastic effects. Any amount of radiation, no matter how small, has the potential to cause harm.

Computed Tomography: Physics and Technology A Self Assessment Guide,
Second Edition. Euclid Seeram.
© 2022 John Wiley & Sons Ltd. Published 2022 by John Wiley & Sons Ltd.

Stochastic effects also are called *late effects*, since the injury may manifest itself years after exposure. Examples of stochastic effects include cancer and genetic damage. Stochastic effects are considered a risk from exposure to the low levels of radiation used in medical imaging, including CT examinations. On the other hand, *deterministic effects* are those for which the severity of the effect (rather than the probability) increases with increasing radiation dose. There is a threshold dose for these effects. Examples of deterministic effects include skin burns, hair loss, tissue damage, and organ dysfunction. Deterministic effects are also referred to as *early effects* and involve high exposures that are unlikely to occur in diagnostic x-ray imaging.

The overall objective of *radiation protection* is to prevent deterministic effects by ensuring that doses remain well below relevant threshold doses and minimizing the probability of stochastic effects. To accomplish this goal, radiation protection in medical imaging is guided by general frameworks such as those established by the International Commission on Radiological Protection (ICRP) and other national radiation protection organizations. This framework includes the principles of justification, optimization, and dose limits. Optimization is designed to protect the patient from unnecessary radiation by using a dose that is considered as low as reasonably achievable (ALARA). The ultimate goal of optimization is to minimize stochastic effects and prevent deterministic effects.

CT dosimetry is complex and characterized by several metrics, such as the *computed tomography dose index* (CTDI), the *dose-length product* (DLP), and the *effective dose*. While the CTDI and DLP are expressed in *milligrays* (mGy), the effective dose is expressed in *millisieverts* (mSv). The effective dose relates radiation exposure to risk and is considered the best method to estimate stochastic radiation risk. Only the first two metrics will be described here.

The *CTDI* is a standardized measure of the radiation dose output of a CT scanner that allows the user to compare the radiation outputs of different CT scanners. It provides a measurement of the exposure per slice and information about the amount of radiation used to perform the study. CT vendors are required to provide the $CTDI_{vol}$ values on the CT scanner console. $CTDI_{vol} = CTDI_w/pitch$ ($CTDI_{weighted} = 1/3\ CTDI_{center} + 2/3\ CTDI_{periphery}$).

$CTDI_{vol}$ is the same whether a 1 mm or 100 mm length of tissue has been scanned. The DLP was introduced to offer a much more accurate representation of the dose for a defined length of tissue (L): it provides a measure of the total dose for a CT examination and can be expressed algebraically as DLP = CTDI$_{vol}$/L. DLP is expressed in mGy-cm.

Dose is related to a number of technical factors such as the kV, mAs, noise, pixel size, and slice thickness. Given these technical factors, the dose can be calculated using the following algebraic expression:

$$dose = k \times \frac{intensity \times beam\,energy}{noise^2 \times pixel\,size^3 \times slice\,thickness}$$

This relation shows that:

1. Reducing the noise in an image by a factor of 2 requires an increase in the dose by a factor of 4.
2. Improving the spatial resolution (pixel size) by a factor of 2 requires an increase in the dose by a factor of 8.
3. Decreasing the slice thickness by a factor of 2 requires an increase in the dose by a factor of 2 (keeping the noise constant).
4. Decreasing both slice thickness and pixel size (spatial resolution) by a factor of 2 requires an increase in the dose by a factor of 16 ($2^3 \times 2 = 2 \times 2 \times 2 \times 2$).
5. Increasing the milliamperage and kilovolt peak increases the patient dose proportionally. For example, a two-fold increase in milliamperage increases the dose by a factor of 2. Additionally, doubling the dose requires an increase by the square of the kilovolt peak.

Other important algebraic expressions to pay attention to are as follows

$$dose \propto \frac{1}{pitch}$$

$$noise \propto \frac{1}{T}$$

where T is the slice thickness.

Iterative reconstruction (IR) algorithms have been introduced in CT to address the problems of the filtered back projection (FBP) reconstruction algorithm (which has been used for decades), such as image artifacts and noise, which are commonplace especially in low-dose CT examinations. For example, several studies have shown that IR algorithms can reduce the dose from 30 to 50%.

Finally, a checklist for dose optimization includes checkup items such as those identified and described by Goo (2012) and includes a body-size-adapted CT protocol, tube current modulation, optimal tube voltage at equivalent radiation dose, a longitudinal scan range, repeat scans, scan modes, and noise-reducing image reconstruction algorithms.

Self-Assessment Questions will be based on each of the following Keywords and Concepts

- Dose optimization definition
- Stochastic effects
- Deterministic effects2e
- Objectives of radiation protection
- CT dosimetry
- Computed Tomography Dose Index (CTDI)
- Units of CTDI
- $CTDI_{volume}$
- Dose Length Product (DLP)
- Factors affecting the dose in CT
- Iterative reconstruction

Challenge Questions

Answer the following questions to check your understanding of the materials studied:

True (T)/False (F)

1. Dose optimization takes into consideration the ALARA (As Low as Reasonably Achievable) of the ICRP.
2. The motivation for dose optimization in CT stems from potential stochastic effects due to exposure to high doses of radiation.

3. Stochastic effects are random: that is, the probability of their occurrence depends on the dose received as the dose increases.
4. There is no threshold dose for stochastic effects.
5. Cancer and genetic damage are examples of stochastic effects.
6. Stochastic effects are also referred to as early effects.
7. Deterministic effects are those for which the severity of the effect (rather than the probability) increases with increasing radiation dose.
8. There is a threshold dose for deterministic effects.
9. Deterministic effects are also referred to as late effects.
10. The optimization radiation protection principle of the ICRP requires the operator to adhere to the ALARA philosophy.
11. The CTDI is a standardized measure of the radiation dose output of a CT scanner that allows the user to compare the radiation outputs of different CT scanners.
12. The dose unit of the CTDI is the sievert.
13. $CTDI_{vol} = CTDI_w/pitch$.
14. The DLP provides a measure of the total dose for a CT examination.
15. Improving the spatial resolution (pixel size) by a factor of 2 requires an increase in the dose by a factor of 8.
16. A two-fold increase in milliamperage increases the dose by a factor of 2.
17. Dose is directly proportional to pitch.
18. Noise in CT is directly proportional to the slice thickness.

Multiple Choice

1. Which of the following refers specifically to the dose optimization principle of the ICRP?
   A. The operator must always apply the ALARA philosophy.
   B. The radiologist is responsible for the dose to the patient.
   C. The patient's doctor determines the dose to the patient.
   D. All are correct.
2. Stochastic effects:
   A. Are effects for which the probability of occurrence depends on the dose
   B. Are effects for which the severity of the effect depends on the dose
   C. Have a threshold dose
   D. Are considered late effects of radiation exposure

3. Stochastic effects:
   A. Have a threshold dose
   B. Have no threshold dose
   C. Are referred to as early effects
   D. Include hair loss and skin burns
4. Deterministic effects:
   A. Are those for which the severity of the effect (rather than the probability) increases with increasing radiation dose
   B. Have a threshold dose
   C. Include hair loss and skin burns
   D. All are correct.
5. The goal of radiation protection is:
   A. To prevent deterministic effects by keeping doses well below threshold doses
   B. To minimize stochastic effects
   C. A only
   D. A and B are correct.
6. Which of the following does not relate to CT dose metrics?
   A. Exposure indicator (EI)
   B. CTDI
   C. DLP
   D. Effective dose
7. The total dose for a CT examination is represented by the:
   A. CTDI
   B. DLP
   C. Effective dose
   D. EI
8. The unit of the effective dose is:
   A. mGy
   B. Coulombs per kilogram (C/kg)
   C. mSv
   D. All are correct.
9. The unit of the CTDI is:
   A. mGy
   B. Coulombs per kilogram (C/kg)
   C. mSv
   D. All are correct.
10. Which of the following algebraic expressions is correct?
    A. $CTDI_{vol} = CTDI_w/pitch$
    B. $CTDI_{vol} = CTDI_w + pitch$

C. $CTDI_{vol} = CTDI_w - pitch$

D. $CTDI_{vol} = pitch/CTDI_w$

11. The following algebraic expression can be used to calculate the DLP:

A. $CTDI_{vol}/L$ (where L is the length of the tissue)

B. $CTDI_{vol} + L$

C. $CTDI_{vol} \times L$

D. $L/CTDI_{vol}$

12. Dose is inversely proportional to:

A. $Noise^2$

B. Slice thickness

C. $Pixel\ size^3$

D. All are correct.

13. Dose is directly proportional to:

A. Beam energy and beam intensity

B. $Noise^2$

C. $Pixel\ size^3$

D. Slice thickness

14. Decreasing both slice thickness and pixel size (spatial resolution) by a factor of 2 requires an increase in the dose by a factor of:

A. 16

B. 8

C. 4

D. 2

15. Dose is:

A. Inversely proportional to pitch

B. Directly proportional to pitch

C. Inversely proportional to $pitch^2$

D. Directly proportional to $pitch^2$

16. Which of the following is correct for the relationship between noise and slice thickness?

A. Noise = slice thickness $(T) \times mAs$

B. $Noise = T^2$

C. $Noise \propto 1/T$

D. $Noise \propto 1T^2$

Short Answers

1. What is the ICRP principle of dose optimization, and why is it important in clinical CT imaging?

2. Explain the difference between stochastic and deterministic effects of radiation exposure, and provide examples of each kind of effect.

3. What is the CTDI?
4. Explain how the $CTDI_{vol}$ is determined
5. What is the DLP? Provide an algebraic expression to calculate it.
6. Explain the relationship between CT dose and beam intensity, beam energy, noise, pixel size, and slice thickness.
7. State the mathematical relationship between dose and pitch, and between CT image noise and slice thickness.
8. Explain the reason for using iterative reconstruction (IR) algorithms, and provide an example of the magnitude of dose reduction using IR algorithms in CT.
9. State the major technical factors that can be used effectively for dose optimization in CT.

Answers to Challenge Questions

True/False

1. T	7. T	13. T
2. T	8. T	14. T
3. T	9. F	15. T
4. T	10. T	16. T
5. T	11. T	17. F
6. F	12. T	18. F

Multiple Choice

1. A	7. B	13. A
2. A	8. C	14. A
3. B	9. A	15. A
4. A	10. A	16. C
5. D	11. A	
6. A	12. D	

Short Answer

1. The ICRP dose optimization principle provides guidance for radiation workers that all exposures must be kept as low as reasonably achievable (ALARA) without compromising the image quality of the examination. Image quality must be diagnostic in order to interpret the patient's medical condition shown in the image. This principle is an integral component of radiation protection

and provides guidance to all operators working in medical imaging as a means of protecting the patient from radiation.

2. Radiation bioeffects are placed in two categories: stochastic effects and deterministic effects. Stochastic effects are those for which the probability of occurrence increases with increasing dose and for which there is no threshold dose. Examples include cancer, leukemia, and hereditary effects. On the other hand, deterministic effects are those for which severity increases with increasing dose and for which there is a threshold dose. Examples include epilation, erythema, and cataracts. These effects provide the motivation for dose optimization.

3. The CTDI is a standardized measure of the radiation dose output of a CT scanner that allows the user to compare the radiation outputs of different CT scanners. The dose unit for the CTDI is the sievert. Knowing the weighted CTDI ($CTDI_w$), the $CTDI_{vol}$ can be calculated using the following algebraic expression:

$$CTDI_{vol} = CTDI_w/pitch$$

4. $CTDI_w = 1/3\ CTDI_{center} + 2/3\ CTDI_{periphery.}$

5. The DLP provides a measure of the total dose for a CT examination and can be expressed algebraically as $DLP = CTDI_{vol}/L$. The DLP is expressed in mGy-cm.

6. The CT dose is directly proportional to the x-ray beam intensity and x-ray beam energy and inversely proportional to the slice thickness, pixel size[3], and noise[2].

7. The CT dose is inversely proportional to the pitch. Increasing the pitch decreases the dose; however, the image quality will be compromised. Noise in CT is inversely proportional to the slice thickness. The thinner the slice, the more noise in the image.

8. Limitations of the FBP algorithm include noise and artifacts in low-dose CT examinations. These limitations are overcome using IR algorithms in low-dose CT imaging. It is reported that IR algorithms can reduce the dose to the patient from 30 to 50%, for example. Currently, all CT vendors offer IR algorithms for their CT scanners.

9. The major technical factors that can be used effectively for dose optimization in CT and described by Dr. Goo (2012) are body size-adapted, CT protocol, tube current modulation, optimal tube voltage at equivalent radiation dose, longitudinal scan range, repeat scans, scan modes, and IR algorithms.

IDENTIFYING AREAS TO STUDY

A. Make a list of topics and/or questions that are still not clear to you after studying this chapter.

B. See the instructor for clarification and/or consolidation of the material.

11

CT Quality Control for Technologists/ Radiographers

PRIOR READING ASSIGNMENT

Before attempting to answer these review questions, read the following brief summary notes of the essentials of quality control in CT.

Quality control (QC) is a subset of quality assurance (QA). While QA deals specifically with the administration of all efforts to ensure that the final products – image quality and the safety of patients and staff in the radiology department from radiation – are of high quality, QC addresses the technical aspects of a QA program. QC is a program that examines and tests the performance of a CT scanner. The goal of a QC program is to ensure that every image created by the CT scanner is a quality image, with minimum radiation dose to patients and personnel. QA and QC are intended to improve the interpretation of images to ensure the correct diagnosis and enhance the quality of patient care.

Computed Tomography: Physics and Technology A Self Assessment Guide,
Second Edition. Euclid Seeram.
© 2022 John Wiley & Sons Ltd. Published 2022 by John Wiley & Sons Ltd.

The essential steps in a QC program have been described in the literature (see Bushong 2021). In particular, QC for CT scanners has been described by organizations such as the International Atomic Energy Agency (IAEA), the American College of Radiology (ACR), the National Council on Radiation Protection and Measurements (NCRP), and the Radiation Protection Bureau – Health Canada (RPB-HC). Fundamentally, QC involves at least three steps: acceptance testing, conducting performance tests and evaluation on a routine basis, and error correction. *Acceptance testing* verifies compliance – that is, whether the CT equipment meets the manufacturer's specifications – and may include verification of slice thickness, CT number linearity, uniformity, spatial and contrast resolution, noise, and dose output. *Routine performance tests and evaluation* include monitoring the components of the CT scanner that affect dose and image quality at specified frequencies (daily, weekly, monthly, or annually). Finally, *error correction* examines the results of the QC tests. If the CT scanner fails to meet the *tolerance limits* or *acceptance limits,* corrective action must be taken to ensure that tolerance limits are met (the scanner must be serviced). These tolerance limits are obtained objectively and are stated by the radiology organizations mentioned earlier. A tolerance limit in QC testing indicates a performance standard range of values that indicates what performance results are within certain tolerances.

Generally, as defined by the organizations mentioned, QC tests are performed on a *daily, weekly, monthly*, and *yearly* basis. Technologists/radiographers play an important role in conducting QC monitoring; however, several tests require the expertise of a medical physicist. The ACR, the IAEA, and Health Canada often prescribe specific tests that should be done by the technologist/radiographer and those that should be done by a qualified medical physicist (QMP). For example, the ACR suggests that the following four tests be done by the CT technologist: CT number for water and standard deviation (noise), artifact evaluation, display monitor QC, and visual inspection of certain components of the scanner.

The IAEA suggests that a QMP should conduct the following tests: CT image quality and radiation protection considerations for the patient, personnel, and members of the public; acquisition and installation of CT scanners, including shielding considerations; and dose optimization.

Conducting CT QC tests requires special equipment and phantoms. The IAEA places these tools in three categories: *image performance phantoms*, *geometric phantoms*, and *quantitative/dosimetry phantoms and instrumentation* (phantoms designed specifically to measure various parameters for QC testing). Furthermore, the ACR recommends using a special phantom referred to as the *ACR accreditation phantom* in its CT accreditation program. This phantom is based on solid water construction and consists of four modules intended to measure positioning accuracy, CT number accuracy, slice thickness, light accuracy alignment, low-contrast resolution, CT number uniformity, and high-contrast resolution. Other phantoms are available from CT vendors as well.

CT QC testing includes at least three basic tenets: QC tests must be done regularly, results must be interpreted promptly, and good and accurate records must be kept.

There are several QC tests for CT scanners, some of which were mentioned earlier. It is not within the scope of this chapter to describe these tests, and therefore the reader must refer to the literature for further details. Three important and routine tests that will be summarized here: the *average CT number for water* (also referred to as the *CT number calibration*, conducted daily), the *standard deviation of the CT numbers in water* (measures *noise* and is also conducted daily), and the *gray-level assessment of the CT image display monitor* (conducted monthly).

The CT calibration test is conducted with a water phantom that is scanned using typical exposure factors. A region of interest (ROI) is placed in the center of the image, and the average CT number for water is measured. It should be 0. Additionally, the ROI is placed outside the image, representing air. The CT number for air is measured, and it should be −1000 if the scanner is properly calibrated. The tolerance limits are set by the country's authority. For example, the IAEA has established a limit of 0 ± 5 HU (Hounsfield units) for the CT number for water, while the limits set by the ACR and the RPB-HC are 0 ± 7 HU and 0 ± 4 HU, respectively.

The standard deviation of the CT number QC test can be done using the same image of the CT number for the water test. The ROI is placed in the center of the image, and the standard deviation of the CT number is measured. This number should be very small. As noted by the ACR, the "limit criteria for the noise (standard deviation) values are primarily determined by the scan technique (radiation dose) used to acquire the images. If the QMP elects to use the manufacturer's specified standard deviation as the limit criteria, the scan technique must be identical to the manufacturer's recommendation (including reconstructed image thickness and reconstruction kernel or filter)."

The gray-level assessment of the CT image display monitor is usually conducted using a test pattern specifically designed for this purpose. One popular such pattern is the SMPTE (Society of Motion Picture and Television Engineers) test pattern, shown in Figure 11.1. The ACR states that "The visual impression should indicate an even progression of gray levels around the 'ring' of gray level patches. Verify

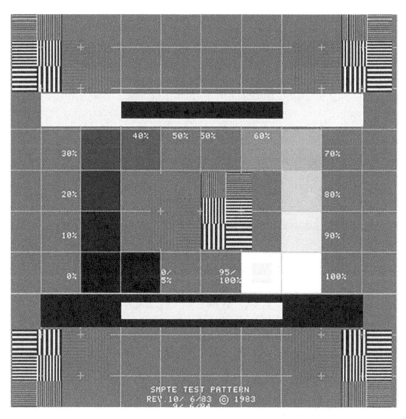

Figure 11.1   Image of the SMPTE test pattern used for gray level assessment of the CT image display monitor.

the following: a) the 5% patch can be distinguished in the 0/5% patch; b) the 95% patch can be distinguished in the 95/100% patch; and c) all the gray level steps around the ring of gray levels are distinct from adjacent steps (note that there are two adjacent squares that are both labelled as 50% which should appear to be equivalent). If these conditions are not met, do not adjust the display window width/level in an effort to correct the problem. Corrective action for the monitor is needed."

Self-Assessment Questions will be based on each of the following Keywords and Concepts

- Quality assurance
- Quality control
- Goal of QC
- Acceptance testing
- Routine testing
- Error correction
- Tolerance or acceptance limits
- IAEA
- ACR
- RPB-HC
- Phantoms for QC testing
- Frequency of QC testing
- Basic tenets of QC testing
- CT number calibration test
- Standard deviation of the CT numbers in water (measures noise)
- Gray-level assessment of the CT image display
- SMPTE test pattern

Challenge Questions

Answer the following questions to check your understanding of the materials studied:

True (T)/False (F)

1. CT QC testing refers to the routine monitoring of the performance of the CT scanner and is concerned with the technical aspects of the equipment.

2. QA refers to the administration of the overall quality management of the equipment in a radiology department and is concerned mainly with people.

3. The overall goal of QC testing is to monitor the performance of operators (technologists, radiographers, and radiologists).

4. The essential steps in QC are acceptance testing, routine testing, and error correction.

5. Acceptance testing verifies compliance: that is, whether the CT scanner meets the manufacturer's specifications.

6. Routine testing refers to the daily assessment of the performance of the scanner.

7. The frequency of QC tests is defined for tests that should be done daily, weekly, monthly, quarterly, bi-annually, and annually.

8. A tolerance limit in QC testing indicates a performance standard range of values that indicates what performance results are within certain tolerances.

9. If a QC test shows that the results are outside the performance range, the scanner must be serviced immediately.

10. Examples of acceptance tests include verification of slice thickness, CT number linearity, uniformity, spatial and contrast resolution, noise, and dose output.

11. The IAEA, the ACR, and the RPB-HC have all issued tolerance limits for various QC tests for CT scanners.

12. The SMPTE test pattern is used to assess the accuracy of CT numbers in the image.

Multiple Choice

1. Which of the following is concerned with monitoring the performance of the CT scanner?
   A. QA
   B. QC
   C. SMPTE test pattern
   D. The geometric CT phantom

2. The administration component of a QC program is referred to as:
   A. QA
   B. Finance
   C. Test tools used in a QC program
   D. Recordkeeping of all QC tests

3. The overall goal of a QC program is to:
   A. Ensure that every image created by the CT scanner is a quality image
   B. Minimize the radiation dose to patients
   C. Minimize the dose to personnel
   D. All are correct.

4. The following are essential steps of a QC program *except*:
   A. The ACR QC phantom
   B. Acceptance testing
   C. Routine performance assessment
   D. Error correction

5. In a QC program, the following is used to verify compliance – that is, whether the CT equipment meets the manufacturer's specifications:
   A. Error correction
   B. Routine testing
   C. Acceptance testing
   D. All are correct.

6. Which of the following is intended to assess whether a CT scanner passes or fails QC tests?
   A. Routine QC monitoring
   B. Acceptance testing
   C. Error correction
   D. Tolerance limits

7. The following performance standard range of values shows whether the results of a QC test should be accepted:
   A. Tolerance limits
   B. Acceptance limits
   C. Scan speed limits
   D. A and B are correct.

8. The IAEA recommends that the QMP conduct this QC test:
   A. Gray-level assessment of the CT display monitor
   B. CT number calibration
   C. Dose optimization
   D. Standard deviation of the CT number for water (noise)

9. The ACR CT QC accreditation phantom is designed to assess:
   A. Positioning accuracy and CT number accuracy
   B. Slice thickness, light accuracy alignment, and low-contrast resolution
   C. CT number uniformity and high-contrast resolution
   D. All are correct.

10. Which is not a basic tenet of CT QC testing?
    A. QC tests must be done on a regular basis.
    B. Results must be interpreted promptly.
    C. The performance of the operator should be checked.
    D. Good and accurate records should be kept.
11. The tolerance limit for the CT number for water as set by the IAEA is:
    A. 0 ± 5 HU
    B. 0 ± 7 HU
    C. 0 ± 4 HU
    D. 0 ± 2 HU
12. The gray-level assessment of the CT image display monitor can be done using the:
    A. ACR QC accreditation phantom
    B. SMPTE test pattern.
    C. Line pair test pattern
    D. All are correct.

Short Answers

1. What is CT QC, and what are the goals of QC?
2. What are the basic tenets of QC?
3. Describe the three essential steps of a QC program.
4. State the types of QC phantoms used for CT QC.
5. Describe the ACR CT QC accreditation program.
6. What are the four CT QC tests for technologists/radiographers recommended by the ACR?
7. Briefly describe the CT QC tests for the CT number for water and the gray-level assessment of the CT scanner display monitor.

Answers to Challenge Questions

True/False

1. T	5. T	9. T
2. T	6. F	10. T
3. F	7. T	11. T
4. T	8. T	12. F

Multiple Choice

1. B	5. C	9. D
2. A	6. A	10. C
3. D	7. D	11. A
4. A	8. C	12. B

Short Answers

1. CT QC is a program that addresses the performance of the technical components of the CT scanner by conducting various tests that require a systematic approach. The overall goal of a CT QC program is to ensure that every image created by the CT scanner is a quality image while at the same time using the minimum radiation dose to create the image. By virtue of this approach, the QC program ensures radiation protection not only for patients but also for personnel. QA and QC are intended to improve the interpretation of images to ensure correct diagnosis and enhance the quality of patient care.

2. There are at least three fundamental tenets of QC:
   A. QC tests must be done regularly.
   B. The results must be interpreted promptly.
   C. There should be good and accurate recordkeeping.

3. The three essential steps in a QC program are acceptance testing, routine performance testing, and error correction. Acceptance testing focuses *on* verifying compliance: that is, whether the CT equipment meets the manufacturer's specifications. It may include verification of slice thickness, CT number linearity, uniformity, spatial and contrast resolution, noise, and dose output, for example. Routine performance testing refers to monitoring the technical components of the CT scanner that affect dose and image quality. These tests are categorized based on whether they should be done daily, weekly, monthly, semi-annually, or annually. Finally, error correction examines the results of the QC tests. If the CT scanner fails to meet the tolerance limits or acceptance limits, then corrective action must be taken to ensure that tolerance limits are met (the scanner must be serviced). A tolerance limit indicates a performance standard range of values that indicates what performance results are within certain tolerances. These limits are obtained objectively and issued by various organizations such as the IAEA, ACR, NCRP, and RPB-HC.

4. Several types of phantoms are used in CT QC programs to test a wide range of technical parameters. Phantoms are usually provided by the CT vendor when the scanner is purchased. The IAEA has placed these phantoms in three categories: image performance phantoms, geometric phantoms, and quantitative/dosimetry phantoms and instrumentation. Additionally, the ACR recommends using a special ACR accreditation phantom for use in its CT accreditation program. This phantom is based on solid water construction and consists of four modules that measure positioning accuracy, CT number accuracy, slice thickness, light accuracy alignment, low-contrast resolution, CT number uniformity, and high-contrast resolution.

5. The ACR phantom is based on solid water construction and consists of four modules intended to measure positioning accuracy, CT number accuracy, slice thickness, light accuracy alignment, low-contrast resolution, CT number uniformity, and high-contrast resolution. This phantom is used in the ACR CT QC accreditation program.

6. In its special CT QC manual, the ACR indicates that the following four tests should be done by the CT technologist:

   A. CT number for water and standard deviation (noise)
   B. Artifact evaluation
   C. Gray-level assessment of the CT image display monitor
   D. Visual inspection of certain components of the scanner

7. The QC test that measures the CT number for water is also referred to as the *CT calibration test*. The following steps are noteworthy:

   1. A water phantom is scanned using typical exposure factors.
   2. A ROI is placed in the center of the image, and the average CT number for water is measured. It should be 0.
   3. The ROI is placed outside the image, representing air, and should have a CT number equal to -1000 (if the scanner is properly calibrated).
   4. The tolerance limits are set by the country's authority. For example, the IAEA has established a limit of $0\pm5\,HU$ (Hounsfield units) for the CT number for water, while the limits set by the ACR and the RPB-HC are 0 ± 7 HU and 0 ± 4 HU, respectively.

The gray-level assessment of the CT image monitor is usually done using the SMPTE image test pattern (or other relevant pattern). This pattern is shown in Figure 11.1. The ACR states that when visually looking at the image of this pattern, two points must be seen in the gray-level assessment:

- The 5% patch can be clearly seen in the 0/5% patch.
- The 95% patch can be clearly seen in the 95/100% patch.

IDENTIFYING AREAS TO STUDY

A. Make a list of topics and/or questions that are still not clear to you after studying this chapter.

B. See the instructor for clarification and/or consolidation of the material.

12

Practice CT Examination: Physics and Technology

1. The first clinically useful CT scanner was developed by:
   A. Cormack
   B. Tsien
   C. Hounsfield
   D. General Electric Company
2. The radiation used by two pioneers in the first CT experiments was:
   A. Gamma rays
   B. X-rays
   C. Beta particles
   D. Cosmic rays
3. What contribution did Cormack make to the development of clinical CT?
   A. He developed Britain's first business computer.
   B. He formulated a program to calculate radiation doses.
   C. He developed mathematical solutions to solve the problem in CT.
   D. He performed practical reconstruction of images from the sun.
4. The major purpose of a spiral/helical CT multislice scanner compared to its conventional slice-by-slice counterpart is to:
   A. Improve the volume coverage speed while maintaining image quality
   B. Use techniques with higher mA and kVp

Computed Tomography: Physics and Technology A Self Assessment Guide,
Second Edition. Euclid Seeram.
© 2022 John Wiley & Sons Ltd. Published 2022 by John Wiley & Sons Ltd.

C. Help the radiologist make a diagnosis that is 100% accurate
D. Scan difficult patients with ease

$$I_0 \rightarrow \boxed{\mu} \rightarrow I$$
$$\leftarrow x \rightarrow$$

5. With reference to the figure, for a homogeneous beam of radiation, which of the following is correct?
   A. $I = I_0 e^{\mu x}$
   B. $I = I_0 e^{-\mu x}$
   C. $I_0 = I e^{-\mu x}$
   D. $\dfrac{I_0}{I} = e^{-\mu x}$

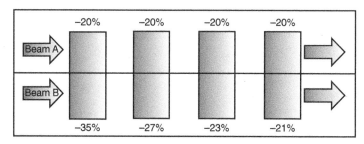

6. From the diagram, which of the following represents a heterogeneous beam of radiation?
   A. A
   B. B

7. In the attenuation of a homogeneous beam of radiation:
   A. The radiation is not attenuated exponentially.
   B. A greater fraction of short wavelengths remains.
   C. There is a change in the quantity of photons.
   D. The beam becomes more penetrating.

8. In the attenuation of a heterogeneous beam of x-rays:
   A. There is a change in x-ray quantity and no change in quality.
   B. The exponential law holds true.
   C. A large portion of low-energy photons remains.
   D. The beam becomes harder or more penetrating.

9. The fractional reduction in the intensity of a beam of radiation per unit thickness of the medium traversed is:
   A. The linear attenuation coefficient
   B. The log of the ratio of the intensity before it enters the medium to the intensity after it transverses the medium

C. The base of the natural logarithm
D. A pixel
10. Which of the following increases radiation attenuation?
    A. Decreasing density
    B. Decreasing the atomic number
    C. Increasing the radiation energy
    D. Decreasing the radiation energy
11. An absorption value of any material within each slice of an object in CT is:
    A. A voxel
    B. The log of the ratio of the intensity of x-rays at the detector to the intensity of x-rays at the source
    C. The log of the ratio of the intensity of x-rays at the source to the intensity of x-rays at the detector
    D. Computed in the digital-to-analog converter
12. Which of the following expressions gives the relationship between CT numbers and the linear attenuation coefficients for tissue (μ_t) and water (μ_w), where K is a scaling factor?

    A. $CT\# = \dfrac{\mu_w - \mu_t}{\mu_t} \bullet K$

    B. $CT\# = K \bullet \dfrac{\mu_t - \mu_w}{\mu_w} \times Euler's\ constant$

    C. $CT\# = \dfrac{\mu_t - \mu_w}{\mu_w} \bullet K$

    D. $CT\# = \dfrac{\mu_t + \mu_w}{\mu_w} \bullet K$

13. The fundamental mathematical problem in CT is to:
    A. Calculate all linear attenuation coefficients (μ) in a specific cross-section given a large set of transmission readings.
    B. Calculate all μs in an object given the scan time and number of detectors.
    C. Calculate all μs in an object cross-section given only the intensity of radiation at the source and the number of detectors.
    D. Calculate all μs given the thickness of the section and the radiation intensity at the detector.

14. What is a RAY SUM within the context of CT?
    A. The sum of the number of x-ray beams and the number of detectors
    B. A transmission measurement along a ray at a given angle
    C. Multiple x-ray beams
    D. The sum of the beams that fall on the detectors

15. In which of the following is the projection data filtered before being back-projected to produce an image that is sharper than one obtained using the back-projection reconstruction technique?
    A. Filtered back projection (also referred to as the convolution method)
    B. Fourier reconstruction
    C. Algebraic reconstruction technique
    D. Iterative least squares technique

16. In terms of speed and accuracy in reconstructing images in CT, which of the following reconstruction algorithms is faster?
    A. Back projection
    B. Filtered back projection
    C. Algebraic reconstruction technique
    D. Iterative least squares method

17. A projection profile is:
    A. The linear attenuation coefficient (μ)
    B. A set of projection data
    C. A ray sum
    D. A beam of x-rays

18. The result of preprocessing the signals from the CT detectors is called:
    A. Convolved data
    B. Reformatted raw data
    C. Image data
    D. Back-projected data

19. The first operation to which reformatted raw data is subjected is referred to as:
    A. Convolution done by the array processors and output as convolved data
    B. Back-projection
    C. 3-D surface rendering
    D. Beam hardening

20. Image data is obtained:
    A. After convolution of the raw data
    B. After preprocessing

    C. After back-projection

    D. Before back-projection

21. Which of the following is subject to back-projection?

    A. Raw data

    B. Convolved data

    C. Reformatted raw data

    D. Image data

22. From which of the following can a diagnosis be made?

    A. Raw data

    B. Reformatted raw data

    C. Image data

    D. Convolved data

23. If the linear attenuation coefficients for bone and water are 0.380 and 0.190, respectively, and the scaling factor of the scanner is 1000, the CT number for bone is:

    A. +1000

    B. −1000

    C. +380

    D. +190

24. The range of CT numbers in an image is called the:

    A. Matrix of the scanner

    B. Window width (WW)

    C. Attenuation coefficient

    D. Window level (WL)

25. The midpoint of a range of CT numbers is the:

    A. WL

    B. WW

    C. Scaling factor

    D. Logarithm of transmission values

26. In CT, a pixel is:

    A. A picture element

    B. A flat surface without thickness

    C. Generally square

    D. All of the above

27. A voxel is:

    A. A picture element on the television monitor

    B. A volume of tissue in the patient

    C. Another term for attenuation coefficient

    D. An absorption value of any material within each slice of the object

28. The contrast of the CT image is essentially controlled by:
   A. A joystick on the scanner
   B. The kVp settings
   C. The mAs used
   D. The window width control

29. An increase in the WL density setting with a fixed WW setting changes the picture from:
   A. Black to white
   B. White to black
   C. No change
   D. Black to brown

30. A window width (WW) of 200 and a window level (WL) of 0 on a CT scanner means that:
   A. Numbers above +100 appear white, numbers below −100 appear black, and the shades of gray extend between +100 and −100.
   B. Numbers below −100 appear white, those above +100 appear black, and the shades of gray extend between +100 and −100.
   C. Numbers above +200 appear black, while those below −200 appear white.
   D. Only numbers above +200 and below −200 appear white and black, respectively.

31.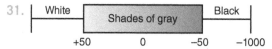

   In the diagram, what are the values of the window width (WW) and window level (WL)?
   A. +1000 and −1000, respectively
   B. +50 and −50, respectively
   C. 100 and 0, respectively
   D. 0 and 0, respectively

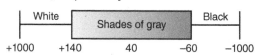

32. In the diagram, what are the values of the WW and WL settings?
   A. 40 and 80, respectively
   B. +140 and −60, respectively

C. 40 and 200, respectively
D. 200 and 40, respectively

White	Shades of gray	Black
+1000	0	−1000

33. In the figure, what is the value of the WW setting if the scale is opened to its maximum and the WL is 0?
   A. +1000
   B. −1000
   C. 0
   D. 2000

34. The purpose of the detector in CT is:
   A. To determine the number of slices to be obtained
   B. To measure the amount of scattered radiation
   C. To measure the x-ray transmission through the patient
   D. All of the above

35. Which of the following determines the thickness of the section to be imaged in CT?
   A. The collimation of the x-ray beam
   B. The pixel width
   C. The technologist
   D. The speed of rotation of the gantry

36. Arrange the following in *increasing order* by CT number:
   1. 1. Air
   2. Bone
   3. Fat
   4. Muscle
   5. Water
      A. 1, 4, 5, 3, 2
      B. 1, 4, 3, 5, 2
      C. 1, 3, 4, 5, 2
      D. 1, 3, 5, 4, 2

37. All of the following can be described as image quality parameters *except*:
   A. Spatial resolution
   B. Low-contrast spatial resolution
   C. Noise
   D. Reconstruction parameters

38. Which of the following describes the scanner's ability to resolve closely spaced objects that are significantly different in the background?
    A. Low-contrast resolution
    B. Spatial resolution
    C. Accuracy
    D. Noise

39. The spatial resolution is specified in terms of:
    A. Line pairs/centimeter (lp/cm)
    B. The number of dark bars seen on the image
    C. The number of white bars seen on the image
    D. The atomic number of the tissue

40. The variation of CT numbers from point to point in the image for a scan of a water phantom is called:
    A. Linearity
    B. Noise
    C. Cross-field uniformity
    D. Contrast resolution

41. For the same FOV, which of the following matrix sizes will result in the smallest pixel size?
    A. 80×80
    B. 256×256
    C. 512×512
    D. 1024×1024

42. What is an indication of a computed tomography system's ability to freeze the motion of the scanned object?
    A. High-contrast resolution
    B. Low-contrast resolution
    C. Spatial resolution
    D. Temporal resolution

43. The area under a typical dose distribution profile for a single scan divided by the slice width is called the:
    A. CTID
    B. MSAD
    C. CTDI
    D. Effective dose

44. The performance characteristics of a CT scanner are tested by:
    A. Quality control procedures
    B. Quality administration policies
    C. Quality care procedures
    D. Management principles of Deming

45. What is the term for the ratio of the difference the table travels per revolution to the width of the beam collimation?
   A. Dose-length product
   B. Pitch ratio
   C. Scan ratio
   D. Tilt ratio

46. The overall goal of volume data acquisition by spiral/helical scanning is to:
   A. Improve image quality
   B. Reduce image artifacts
   C. Increase the volume coverage speed
   D. Reduce the dose to the patient

47. The cable wrap-around problem in conventional CT is resolved by using which of the following?
   A. High-capacity x-ray tube
   B. High-frequency generator
   C. Slip ring technology
   D. Spiral/helical weighting algorithm

48. In spiral/helical CT scanning, an *interpolation algorithm* is needed to:
   A. Produce a planar section (data set).
   B. Reconstruct the final CT image in the volume.
   C. Remove streaking artifacts caused by the presence of metal.
   D. Remove beam hardening artifacts.

49. The purpose of the slip ring in a spiral/helical CT scanner is to:
   A. Remove ring artifacts.
   B. Allow the table to move only 10 cm.
   C. Provide continuous rotation of the x-ray tube and detectors so that a volume of tissue can be scanned.
   D. Provide increased voltage to the x-ray tube.

50. For spiral/helical CT scanning, which of the following pitch ratios produces the best image quality?
   A. 1 : 1
   B. 2 : 1
   C. 3 : 1
   D. 6 : 1

51. Which of the following pitch ratios will result in the largest volume coverage in the fastest time?
   A. 1:1
   B. 2:1
   C. 4:1
   D. 6:1

52. One of the most noticeable differences between single-slice and multislice CT systems is the:
   A. Detector design
   B. Computer system
   C. Image display subsystem
   D. Thickness of the section

53. For multislice CT scanning, the size of the slice is determined by:
   A. The number of channels in the detector design
   B. The DAS
   C. The number of detector elements grouped together (binned)
   D. All of the above

54. In spiral/helical CT scanning, which of the following is the *effective mAs*?
   A. Effective mAs = kilovolts/pitch
   B. Effective mAs = mAs + pitch
   C. Effective mAs = mAs/pitch
   D. Effective mAs = pitch/kilovolts

55. The definition of pitch ratio in a multislice scanner, as defined by the International Electrotechnical Commission, states that:
   A. P = distance the table travels per rotation (d)/total collimation (W)
   B. P = d + W
   C. P = d×W
   D. P = W/d

56. When all sides of a voxel are equal (perfect cube), the data acquired in CT is said to be:
   A. Anisotropic
   B. Dystrophic
   C. Isotropic
   D. Unitropic

57. The QC test for the average CT number for water should be done:
   A. Daily
   B. Weekly
   C. Monthly
   D. Annually

58. The tolerance limit for the QC test for the average CT number for *water* from SC-35 is:
    A. 0±5 CT numbers
    B. 0±4 CT numbers
    C. 0±1 CT number
    D. 0–1

59. The tolerance limit for the QC test for the CT number for *air* is:
    A. −1000±10 CT numbers
    B. 1000±3 CT numbers
    C. 100±1 CT number
    D. +1000±10 CT numbers

60. The tolerance limit for a computed tomography number calibration quality control test, as stated by the IAEC, is:
    A. 0±5 HU
    B. 10±5 HU
    C. 0±8 HU
    D. No tolerance limit has been established as yet.

References

Bushong, S. (2021). *Radiologic Science for Technologists*, 12e. St Louis, MO: Mosby-Elsevier.

Goo, H.W. (2012). CT radiation dose optimization and estimation: an update for radiologists. *Korean Journal of Radiology* 13 (1): 1–11. https://doi.org/10.3348/kjr.2012.13.1.1.

Leng, S., Bruesewitz, M., Tao, S. et al. (2019). Photon-counting detector CT: system design and clinical applications of an emerging technology. *Radiographics* 39: 729–743. https://doi.org/10.1148/rg.2019180115.

Seeram, E. (2018). *CT at a Glance*. Oxford, UK: Wiley.

Seeram, E. (2020). Computed tomography image reconstruction. *Radiol. Technol.* 92 (2): 155CT–169CT. PMID: 33203780.

FURTHER READING

Barrett, J.F. and Keat, N. (2004). Artifacts in CT: recognition and avoidance. *Radiographics* 24 (6): 1679–1691. https://doi.org/10.1148/rg.246045065.

Baxes, G.A. (1994). *Digital Image Processing: Principles and Applications*. New York: Wiley.

Beister, M., Kolditz, D., and Kalender, W.A. (2012). Iterative reconstruction methods in x-ray CT. *Phys. Med.* 28 (2): 94–108. https://doi.org/10.1016/j.ejmp.2012.01.003.

Berrington de Gonzalez, A., Mahesh, M., Kim, K.P. et al. (2009, 2009). Projected cancer risks from computed tomographic scans performed in the United States in 2007. *Arch. Intern. Med.* 169 (22): 2071–2077. https://doi.org/10.1001/archintern med.2009.440.

Bushberg, J.T., Seibert, J.A., Leidholdt, E.M., and Boone, J.M. (2021). *The Essential Physics of Medical Imaging*, 4e. Philadelphia, PA: Lippincott Williams & Wilkins.

Government of Canada (2008). Safety code 35: Safety procedures for installation, use and control of x-ray equipment in large medical radiological facilities. https://www.canada.ca/en/health-canada/services/environmental-workplace-health/reports-publications/radiation/safety-code-

35-safety-procedures-installation-use-control-equipment-large-medical-radiological-facilitiessafety-code.html (accessed 8 November 2021).

Hricak, H., Brenner, D.J., Adelstein, S.J. et al. (2011). Managing radiation use in medical imaging: a multifaceted challenge. *Radiology* 258 (3): 889–905. https://doi.org/10.1148/radiol.10101157.

Hsieh, J. (2008). *Adaptive Statistical Iterative Reconstruction*. Whitepaper, GE Healthcare.

IEC (1999). *Medical Electrical Equipment-60601 Part 2-44: Particular Requirements for the Safety of x-ray Equipment for CT*. Geneva, Switzerland: International Electrotechnical Commission.

Image Gently. (2021) www.imagegently.com (accessed 26 November 2021).

Kalender, W. (2005). *Computed Tomography Fundamentals, System Technology, Image Quality, Applications*. Erlangen, Germany: Publicis Corporate Publishing.

Kaza, R.K., Platt, J.F., Goodsitt, M.M. et al. (2014). Emerging techniques for dose optimization in abdominal CT. *Radiographics* 34 (1): 4–17. https://doi.org/10.1148/rg.341135038.

Mutic, S., Palta, J.R., Butker, E.K. et al. (2003). Quality assurance for CT simulators and CT simulation process. Report of the AAPM radiation therapy committee task group No 66. *Med. Phys.* 30: 2762–2792. https://doi.org/10.1118/1.1609271.

Qiu, D. and Seeram, E. (2016). Does iterative reconstruction improve image quality and reduce dose in computed tomography? *Radiol Open J.* 1 (2): 42–54. https://doi.org/10.17140/ROJ-1-108.

Seeram, E. (2014). Computed tomography dose optimization. *Radiol. Technol.* 85 (6): 655CT–671CT.

Seeram, E. (2022). *Computed Tomography: Physical Principles, Clinical Applications, and Quality Control*. Philadelphia, PA: Saunders Elsevier (in Press).

Seeram, E. and Brennan, P.C. (2006). Diagnostic reference levels in radiology. *Radiol. Technol.* 77 (5): 373–384.

Seeram, E. and Seeram, D. (2008). Image postprocessing in digital radiology: a primer for technologists. *J. Med. Imaging Radiat. Sci.* 39 (1): 23–41. https://doi.org/10.1016/j.jmir.2008.01.004.

Seibert, J.A. (2014). Iterative reconstruction: how it works, how to apply it. *Pediatr. Radiol.* 44 (suppl 3): 431–439. https://doi.org/10.1007/s00247-014-3102-1.

Shefer, E., Altman, A., Behling, R. et al. (2013). State of the art of CT detectors and sources: a literature review. *Curr. Radiol. Rep.* 1 (1): 76–91. https://doi.org/10.1007/s40134-012-0006-4.

Ulzheimer, S. and Kappler, S. (2017). Photon-counting detectors in clinical computed tomography. https://health.siemens.com/ct_applications/somatomses sions/index.php/photon-counting-detectors-in-clinical-computed-tomography/ (accessed 8 November 2021).

Appendix A
Answers to CT
Review Questions

1. C	21. B	41. D
2. A	22. C	42. D
3. C	23. A	43. C
4. A	24. B	44. A
5. B	25. A	45. B
6. B	26. D	46. C
7. C	27. B	47. C
8. D	28. D	48. A
9. A	29. B	49. C
10. D	30. A	50. A
11. C	31. C	51. D
12. C	32. D	52. A
13. A	33. D	53. C
14. B	34. C	54. C
15. A	35. A	55. A
16. B	36. D	56. C
17. B	37. D	57. A
18. B	38. B	58. B
19. B	39. A	59. A
20. C	40. B	60. A

Computed Tomography: Physics and Technology A Self Assessment Guide,
Second Edition. Euclid Seeram.
© 2022 John Wiley & Sons Ltd. Published 2022 by John Wiley & Sons Ltd.

Index

Page locators in *italics* indicate figures. This index uses letter-by-letter alphabetization

Computed Tomography: Physics and Technology A Self Assessment Guide, Second Edition. Euclid Seeram.
© 2022 John Wiley & Sons Ltd. Published 2022 by John Wiley & Sons Ltd.